TAO OF LETTING GO

Other Books by Bruce Frantzis

Relaxing into Your Being (Tao Meditation, Volume 1):
Chi, Breathing and Dissolving Inner Pain

The Great Stillness (Tao Meditation, Volume 2):
Body Awareness, Moving Meditation and Sex Qigong

Chi Revolution:
Harness the Healing Power of Your Life Force

Opening the Energy Gates of Your Body:
Qigong for Lifelong Health

The Power of Internal Martial Arts and Chi:
Combat and Energy Secrets of Ba Gua, Tai Chi and Hsing-I

Tai Chi: Health for Life:
Why It Works for Health, Stress Relief and Longevity

Dragon and Tiger Medical Qigong:
Health and Energy in Seven Simple Movements

Bagua and Tai Chi:
Exploring the Potential of Chi, Martial Arts, Meditation and the I Ching

Taoist Sexual Meditation:
The Way of Love, Energy and Spirit

TAO OF LETTING GO
MEDITATION FOR MODERN LIVING

Bruce Frantzis

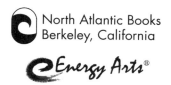

North Atlantic Books
Berkeley, California

Energy Arts®

Tao of Letting Go: Meditation for Modern Living

Published by Energy Arts, Inc. Publications, P. O. Box 99, Fairfax, CA 94978
Distributed by North Atlantic Books, P. O. Box 12327, Berkeley, CA 94712

The following trademarks are used under license by Energy Arts, Inc., from Bruce Frantzis: Frantzis Energy Arts® system, Mastery Without Mystery®, Longevity Breathing® program, Opening the Energy Gates of Your Body™ Qigong, Marriage of Heaven and Earth™ Qigong, Bend the Bow™ Spinal Qigong, Spiraling Energy Body™ Qigong, Gods Playing in the Clouds™ Qigong, Living Taoism™ collection, Chi Rev Workout™, HeartChi™ and ℰ *Energy Arts* ®

North Atlantic Books is part of the Society for the Study of Native Arts and Sciences, a nonprofit educational corporation whose goals are to develop an educational and cross-cultural perspective linking various scientific, social and artistic fields; to nurture a holistic view of arts, sciences, humanities and healing; and to publish and distribute literature on the relationship of mind, body and nature.

Editing: Heather Hale, Energy Arts, Inc., and Anne Connolly, North Atlantic Books, Inc.
Interior Design: Lisa Petty, GirlVibe, Inc.
Cover Design: Rick Snizik, Snizik Marketing and Design, LLC.
Copyediting: Nancy Riccio, Plateau MediaWorks, Inc.
Illustrations: Michael McKee
Back Cover Photo: Richard Marks

Printed in the United States of America

PLEASE NOTE: The practice of Taoist energy arts and the meditative arts may carry risks. The information in this book is not in any way intended as a substitute for medical, psychological or emotional counseling with a licensed physician or healthcare provider. The reader should consult a professional before undertaking any martial arts, movement, meditative arts, health or exercise program to reduce the chance of injury or any other harm that may result from pursuing or trying any technique discussed in this book. Any physical or other distress experienced during or after any exercise should not be ignored and should be brought to the attention of a healthcare professional. The creators and publishers of this book disclaim any liabilities for loss in connection with following any of the practices described in this book, and implementation is at the discretion, decision and risk of the reader.

Library of Congress Cataloging-in-Publication Data

Frantzis, Bruce Kumar.
  The tao of letting go : how to meditate / Bruce Frantzis.
    p. cm.
  ISBN 978-1-55643-808-0
  1. Meditation--Taoism. I. Title.
  BL1923.F74 2009
  299.5'14435--dc22

2 3 4 5 6 7 8 9 Peter Schultz Printing 17 16 15 14 13 12

CONTENTS

DEDICATION

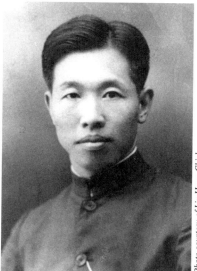

Photo courtesy of Liu Hung Chieh

Liu Hung Chieh in his early twenties.

This book is a culmination of all of the knowledge of chi I have acquired in more than forty years as a martial artist, chi master, Taoist priest and energetic healer.

I thank all my teachers through the years, including my last and primary teacher, the late Taoist Lineage Master, Liu Hung Chieh of Beijing, who took in a Westerner and taught him the secrets of chi, which had been closely guarded for millennia. It is with my deepest gratitude that I extend to you this information to do my part to make the world a better place.

ACKNOWLEDGMENTS

I would like to express my sincere gratitude to Liu Hung Chieh who passed down his Taoist meditation lineage to me.

Although several people helped in the actual creation of this book, special appreciation for editing and project management goes to Heather Hale, Director, Energy Arts, Inc.

I'd also like to thank Anne Connolly at North Atlantic Books for developmental editing; Teja Bell for writing the foreword; Lisa Petty, GirlVibe, Inc., for interior design and production; Richard Snizik, Snizik Marketing and Design, LLC, for the cover design; Nancy Riccio, Plateau MediaWorks, for copyediting; Michael McKee for illustrations; and Richard Marks for the back cover photograph.

Finally, deep appreciation goes to my wife Caroline for her copyediting and her never-ending inspiration and support.

FOREWORD

You have in your hands a book that can transform your life. Its teachings are based on ancient Taoism. Yet they are relevant to our times and circumstances and are voiced in a language that is both accessible and deep. Even in

> *"When I let go of what I am, I become what I might be."*
> – Lao Tse

retreats and centers where Buddhist practice is the guiding endeavor, I find that when I offer the Taoist dissolving practices that are presented here, they resonate deeply with meditators. Taoists are known for their practicality. Whatever is practical is also useful. *Tao of Letting Go* is practical teaching at its best. The usefulness of the teachings directly touches on what is important and even necessary to our well-being in the areas of body, mind, emotions and ultimately expressing our true nature.

The practices presented in *Tao of Letting Go* bring to life the ancient teachings of the masters of the Tao. As you explore the Personal Practice Sessions and the Author-guided Practice Sessions presented throughout the book or the audio set, you may come to directly know ancient wisdom, not as an arcane teaching, but as your own present knowing. This direct knowing is, in fact, the purpose and the direction of all meditation practices in all traditions. There can be no more simple equation than: do the practice—experience freedom. While the practices are simple, they are not simplistic. Simplicity is the gateway to depth for those who are willing to give their attention with patience to practice.

As a teacher of meditation and qigong, I have presented these practices to my students for more than a decade. Effective for creating internal freedom, the Inner Dissolving method and its many variations and applications are transformative and powerful. My students connect immediately with an embodied experience of release, or letting go into the present—freeing the hinges of identification with

> *"I have just three things to teach: simplicity, patience, compassion. These three are your greatest treasures."*
>
> — Lao Tse

emotional, mental or physical trauma that tend to continue the cycles of suffering. More so, the "field" of well-being that ripples out of these practices positively impacts the interconnected emotional, mental and physical "bodies." Letting go into the present is the place where all true healing takes place. As you work with the wisdom presented here, *letting go* will become an actualized experience and not a trite aphorism. Be patient. Patience embraces trust. Give yourself the gift of letting go, and in the expression of this true compassion for yourself, you also share this gift with all of life.

Teja Bell, meditation, dharma and qigong teacher at Spirit Rock Meditation Center, Rinzai Lineage Zen Priest

INTRODUCTION

Why Meditate?

In modern life, we are constantly chasing after things in the external world. But you will never find peace in any external object. Any external object you get will eventually become boring and lose its appeal. Meditation is about peace. It's about finding joy and happiness inside yourself.

Many people have internal demons, blockages or obstacles that tear them apart. Meditation can help free you from these demons and from your incessant wants and desires, which keep you spinning like a hamster on a wheel, continually seeking one thing after another. Meditation can eventually bring you a sense of compassion, balance and wisdom.

Meditation can also teach you to let go of that which you probably know you would be better off without. Most people don't really want to hate; most people don't want to be constantly wrenched with anger. Anger in itself is natural, but most of the time it only makes you miserable and poisons your body. Does anybody truly want to be depressed most of the time? Does anybody truly want to have the thoughts in their mind that never stop like an endless carousel that allows no rest? Peace can be extremely difficult to find in this world.

Meditation not only helps you connect to yourself, it also clears out that which prevents you from connecting to others. One of the primary concerns of Taoism is to allow you to connect to the sense of nature and the universe. Look up at the night sky: It's really, really big up there. Most people are inside themselves, imprisoned by their egos. They are not connected to what is deep inside them. In fact, if there has been one common purpose of meditation throughout all of history, it is connecting you to the depth of yourself. Whether you want to call it awakening to your soul, awakening to God, or becoming awake like Buddha, it's all about becoming natural. All of these phrases are about connecting to your innermost core.

When you begin to awaken you find that your capacity and ability to connect to everything slowly increases. If anything is true about this electronic-information age, it's that people are incredibly disconnected. Wisdom and the sense of a connection to reality is not the same thing as little bits and bytes of information floating by. Those are just thoughts, and no matter how true they are, they don't leave you feeling satisfied and fully alive.

The whole process of meditation is about releasing whatever inhibits you. If you can recognize that the way you experience the world is determined by the lens through which you view it, you will realize that getting rid of the obstacles that prevent you from seeing life clearly is the most direct way to becoming happy. You gain a sense of clarity and a sense of connection to everything.

When a human being does not feel connected to the deepest level of their being, they cannot find happiness. Becoming connected is a high art that can make a fool wise.

Meditation allows you to relax at the core of your soul so you can take on the challenging pursuits of finding a sense of balance and having compassion for other beings—the most valuable endeavors you can undertake in this life.

Integrating the Experiences of Your Life

In the modern age there are millions of inputs constantly bombarding us. You can't figure out what is important with so much useless data floating around. The depths of a human being are much more complex. We have wonderful experiences and horrible experiences. We have stress and we have joy. We need to integrate our experiences in order to pull everything together into the core of our being. There has to be some place where you just can let everything settle, where you can simply be a human being at peace with yourself.

In ancient times, when people actually lived by the stars and seasons, they were in tune with the natural rhythms of life. Today endless deadlines, the "hurry up and wait," destroy natural human rhythms.

We rush and push and don't have regular rest and activity cycles, so stress levels rise. A mind that cannot rest slowly goes crazy. A body that does not rest eventually becomes sick. When the body becomes agitated, the mind becomes agitated. A negative feedback loop is created and the body reacts with a full-blown stress response. Over time, you find that you can't sleep and your resting cycles are interrupted. Eventually you lose your emotional stability and seemingly without warning you have emotional outbursts. All of this happens because you have not allowed yourself sufficient time to integrate the experiences of your life to a point where everything goes quiet.

Meditation has been used for thousands of years by every religious tradition to create these rhythms and give people a way of finding peace, balance, compassion and a sense of morality. Monasteries, some of the most structured places for meditation, have a time for work and a time for prayer. They set a rhythm that allows people to fall into deep periods of silence and integrate their experiences. We all have an intrinsic need for this natural rhythm.

Sitting and meditating allows your system to settle so that you can integrate your experiences and connect. These periods of integration help you understand the parts of yourself that are essential to living a smooth, peaceful and happy life. In the process of integrating you begin to recognize what is important and what is not. It may not feel like your everyday life allows for this, but sitting and meditating will help create that space for you.

> *Sitting and meditating allows your system to settle so that you can integrate your experiences and connect.*

What Is Meditation?

People may say they meditate and it sounds wonderful, but you don't know what it is they're really doing. The same goes for people who say they pray. The politically correct response is, "Oh, that's wonderful—you pray." Of course, you don't actually know if they are praying to God, to a particular angel, the devil or even the ice-cream man down the street. Just saying you pray or meditate is supposed to be enough.

There are many forms of meditation, but many people in the West confuse meditation with contemplation. That is, they think about something. If you think about an idea, that's meditating on an idea—as in the meditations of Marcus Aurelius, the famous Roman emperor. From an Eastern point of view, that's not meditation—that's analysis. In the West the subject of meditation gets somehow lumped under the term "philosophy." Philosophers often devote time to thinking about how they think and what it is they should be thinking. Although there is value in considering how we will order our thoughts and what thoughts are truly worthwhile, such activity still cannot be called meditation. It's a form of contemplation—contemplating your thoughts.

When you look deeper, philosophy and meditation are really quite different. Philosophy generally has some ideas about how you are meant to live your life; for example, you shouldn't lie and you should tell the truth. Philosophies dictate the expectations you set for yourself or for someone else. Eastern philosophies have ideas of karma and reincarnation. Western philosophies have ideas of God, heaven and hell.

Meditation is not thinking about something. Meditation is the process of releasing any blocked energy that is attached to any thought. It is about how you can change the deepest substructures of your mind and soul so that you have a way to be happy. Understanding what prevents you from being happy is not enough. You need a method that allows you to get there. Meditation is the ability to let go and change the structure inside of you that drives conscious thought in the first place.

The attitude that you are going to "get something" from meditation is actually the problem that meditation is trying to solve. You will be dissatisfied with meditation as long as your approach is only to obtain something. Save your expectations for buying a car, acquiring money, or planning a vacation; leave expectations out of meditation. The Buddha meditated not to get something but to become free of the need to get something.

Lao Tse's Tradition

The techniques described in this text come from the Water method of Taoist meditation, described by Lao Tse in the *Tao Te Ching* over 2,500 years ago. According to this sophisticated tradition, which has been transmitted for millennia from teacher to disciple in an unbroken lineage to the Taoist sage Liu Hung Chieh and from him to me,[1] spiritual pursuits start with improving the health of the physical body. The practitioner therefore seeks to become relaxed, fully alive and balanced before taking on the more difficult challenges of working with the unseen spirit world.

Balancing Expectations

Another intrinsic aspect of meditation is that it relieves us from the tyranny of expectations. In the modern age people are conditioned to constantly meet external expectations to the point that they don't even know why they have those expectations in the first place. This is not the road to freedom. This is not the road to peace of mind. This is the road to power: I expect something and I do anything I can until I get it.

Expectations have their pros and cons. If you want to take advantage of a world that has marvelous scientific and organizational wonders, then you need expectations. However, in your inner world, most of these expectations put you in direct conflict with yourself—maybe you want to practice, but you find that you are too tired at the end of the day after fulfilling your responsibilities. Maybe you want to show more compassion to others, but, when people upset you, somehow you find yourself losing patience.

---

[1] See the author's book, *The Power of Internal Martial Arts and Chi*, for a detailed account of his training.

Thus the question becomes how to balance your inner world so that you are not overrun by your expectations. What is the result of being driven by expectation? You are never present to what is actually happening to you. Instead you are present in your mind to 10,000 events that happened before, to what events you think should be happening and to what they're going to produce. You are not present to what is actually happening in the moment.

Expectations may be accompanied by a tremendous amount of negativity. If we expect something to be so and it's not, what happens? People turn negative: angry, sad, depressed or disappointed. Meditation has the power to take you towards a more positive view of life. The truth is that most things are neither positive nor negative, but have much more to do with your perspective. Things happen—such is the nature of life. Getting stuck and being unable to move forward is what the world of expectations does to people. Meditation can release you from your incessant wants and desires.

An Education about Your Inner World

Thomas Jefferson used to say that an electorate had to be educated to understand how a democracy functioned. Likewise, those who meditate seek an education about their inner world. Your inner world is how you experience life. It is what determines whether you feel happiness, peace or joy. Meditators through the ages have discovered that you have to learn what is inside you before you can have the faintest clue about whether you are taking care of your inner world.

Going to the depth of your being is the only way you will find wisdom. Meditation is not about giving away your power, but about giving away the

> *Going to the depth of your being is the only way you will find wisdom.*

need to be powerful. The aim is to just be. You flow with life, accepting life as it is. As you let go, the only thing you have left to do is become happier. You simply become at ease with life.

The few books on Taoism available in English tend to use obscure metaphorical language that Westerners find extremely difficult to understand. *Tao of Letting Go* is deliberately presented in a conversational, down-to-earth style to make the potent tradition of Taoist meditation accessible and relevant to modern readers. The aim is to help you go inside yourself and discover the tools to let go, allowing you to adapt more smoothly to the ever-changing conditions of life.

Meditation is the tool. Every genuine meditation tradition since the dawn of time has within it practical methods that have consistently given human beings a way to let go and move from where they are now to where they would like to be. If people knew what they were doing really wasn't working and all they had to do was think about the changes they wanted to make, the world would be a very different place. Thinking about change is not enough. There has to be something that can free up your insides so you become capable of actually making change. First and foremost, this is what meditation is about. If you take your practice far enough you might eventually arrive at the lofty goal of enlightenment, as Buddhists would say, or what contemplative Christians would describe as directly communing with God.

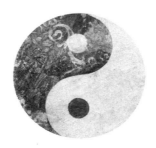

CHAPTER 1
The Water Tradition of Taoist Meditation

Taoism is the original meditation, religion and philosophy of the Chinese. Taoism is naturalistic. One of its main goals is the development of true spontaneity, which has largely been lost in the modern world. The more we live by expectations, the less spontaneous we become. People want to look good on the outside, but they take little care of their internal environment.

Taoists consider human beings to be a part of nature, so first and foremost you must develop a true relationship with yourself. The classic Taoist phrase is "relaxing into your being," into the core of yourself. Taoists don't believe in any gods—or you could say they believe in all gods. The inner meditation tradition of Taoism, having few ceremonies and rituals, is not particularly religious. Taoists are primarily concerned with freeing people from their internal struggles.

Inner versus Outer Wealth

Today a lot of religions proselytize by spreading a gospel of prosperity. Join this religion or church and you will get rich, powerful or whatever it is you want. These groups are addressing the whole issue of outer wealth. But meditation in every genuine tradition makes a core distinction between the external world and your inner life.

An outer life is important. You need to make money, to receive schooling, to have a job and a place to live. All of this can be approached in a fairly practical manner. But your inner life is equally important. What is it inside you that will allow you to ride out the many ups and downs of life? Regardless of external circumstance, how do you cultivate inner wealth? Just as you can build external wealth steadily, you can build your inner world steadily. Happiness is a sense of being connected to everything. It has to come from inside you. Where inside do you find peace? Where do you find stability in your mind?

Even in places where people are the poorest, where life is the hardest, some people have incredible inner turmoil and others are incredibly happy. Material wealth is not necessarily the indicator of happiness. Instead it is what is going on inside you. As people become clear about what is truly inside of them, it follows that they usually become a lot clearer about how to deal with the outer world. Taoist meditation can help you find this clarity.

The Water Tradition

Within Taoism, there are two branches. The Chinese call them Fire and Water, or yang and yin.

The yang or Fire branch is a method of transformation. Through some act of conscious will or effort you seek to create the kind of mind you want. For example, if you have a tape in your head that says you are an utterly horrible person, then you might want to replace it with a tape that says you are really cool. Likewise, if you have a tape in your head that says you will never be okay, then you want to replace it with a tape that says you are okay now and will be forever. This is a path of transformation. The Fire approach to meditation essentially seeks to create some sort of hypnotic state, typically through the use of visualizations, which you may later choose to break down to free yourself from your conditioning.

The yin or Water method aims to release everything that is not real, or relative, so all that remains is what is real, or constant, through whatever circumstances or changes that may occur. If you think you are a terrible person or unworthy of life, you want to have the intent to release that belief. You do this for any belief that prevents you from coming back to your core, where you can be fully awake. When people are awake they are not only comfortable with themselves but they are also happy with existence and the universe.

Balance, Then Compassion

Taoists start with balance in order to later arrive at the lofty goal of compassion. How to find balance between our inner and outer world is a major issue. There is what genuinely feels natural to you and what the whole world is telling you should be natural. In the modern age, where everything is going to extremes, there is a serious lack of balance. So, how do you recognize these extremes and move more toward the middle? This question is at the core of Taoist philosophy and meditation.

The 70 Percent Rule

To achieve balance, Taoists make use of the 70 percent rule, which states that when practicing, you never exceed 70 percent of your ability. This principle applies to all aspects of your practice, including the duration and level of difficulty. I've written extensively about many specifics of the 70 percent rule of moderation in my other books,[1] but the basic concept is that if you avoid extreme behavior—neither doing too little or too much to create any given effect—gradually you get used to being more balanced in your approach to achieving any goal. Along the way, you avoid burnout and you avoid never making progress toward a desired goal because of either pushing too hard or not exerting enough effort. First, you apply this principle to your practice; and eventually you grow your capacity to apply it to all aspects of your life. That which is not sustainable will not continue. Force and, equally, indifference will not help you reach your true potential.

---

[1] See the author's books: *The Chi Revolution*, p. 33; *Tai Chi: Health for Life*, p. 37; and *Opening the Energy Gates of Your Body*, p. 28.

Old View for the New World

The Taoist worldview of how the mind and the spirit work together can be likened to quantum physics, which states that everything is connected to everything else. So the sheer act of observing something changes it.[2] And, central to Taoist philosophy is the premise that all people consist of energy.

When you become fixated on your thoughts, traumas and ideas, you start treating them as though they are real, as if they are solid "objects." Not only do you think these fixations are real, but also you start treating these "objects" as if they are you. You allow them to control you, or maybe you hope they will so you don't actually have to exert any effort of your own. But when you really get right down to it, all your thoughts, emotions and memories are nothing more than energy.

Energy either flows freely or it becomes blocked. When energy is blocked, imbalances emerge and you easily find yourself caught in a cul-de-sac of emotional explosions, churning thoughts and bodily pain, from which there never seems to be an end. The Water method, which was passed down by Lao Tse,[3] asserts that if you become present to what's inside you, you can become aware of what is flowing or blocked.

If your energy is flowing, there's no problem—events seem to come and go naturally. When energy becomes blocked, a cascade of imbalances is set off and you experience pain—whether physical, emotional or mental. For example, if an acupuncture point in the body becomes blocked, you might experience physical pain. That physical pain may link to your emotions and thinking, creating a negative feedback loop that amplifies the effects of that blockage. So when you recognize that an area is blocked, you want to focus your attention on it.

---

[2] See Lynne McTaggart's books, *The Intention Experiment* (Free Press, 2007) and *The Field* (Harper Perennial, 2002).
[3] Author of the *Tao Te Ching*, of which numerous translations are available in English.

If you are present, you can develop the ability to recognize places in your body where energy is blocked. Then you can bring your intention to those places to break up and release the blockages. Research has shown that positive and negative thoughts profoundly affect the healing process all the way down to the cellular level.[4] The Water method does not involve using force to achieve the result you want. Instead you wait until the energy itself, by the use of your attention, somehow connects to what is at the core of that blockage and all of its interconnections—other blockages you may not be aware of or ready to deal with. Then you use your intention to release the blockage.

Accepting the Here and Now

Most people confuse intention with thinking. That is, they try to release blocked energy by following the thoughts in their head. This won't work because of the greatest single issue in the world of psychology: denial. The mind will throw up all kinds of thoughts to distract you from discovering the true source of energy behind those blockages. To further complicate matters, a thought may not necessarily be conscious, but rather energy moving inside you that has a life of its own. Many people cannot deal with problems that sit right in front of them, issues that clearly should be dealt with, because of denial. Until you get to the point where you can recognize what is happening, you might stay with a blockage for a lifetime. When you can recognize and stay with this energy, you can feel what is blocked and eventually release it.

In meditation practice a release and resolution goes through three basic stages: 1) recognizing what is; 2) active waiting for a release of any blockages you have identified; and 3) accepting what is—even if it isn't your ultimate ideal. You may be feeling bad right now; you might be under stress; you might have had a horrible day. Maybe you just want a couple minutes of peace. If you release everything

If you release everything inside you, peace will arise naturally.

---

[4] See *The Biology of Belief* (Mountain of Love Productions and Elite Press, 2005) by Bruce H. Lipton.

inside you, peace will arise naturally. With regular practice, most people find that they can accept and successfully navigate the here and now.

I don't know if you have ever gone for a month or more without taking a shower or a bath, but after a certain point, you really start feeling grimy. Even the worst teenager who never wants to clean up will feel good when he finally takes that bath. Maybe you can go a week or two and not even notice the dirt if you have enough going on, but at some point you are going to feel it. Just as you take baths to cleanse your physical body, you also need to take spiritual baths to clean out your insides. This is what allows you internal space so you can be at peace. You must do some regular cleaning to prevent massive build-up. This is why people in all the classic religious traditions pray, commune or meditate on a regular basis.

The Dissolving Method

If you could grant just one wish to most people who recognize their faults or problems, they would wish for them to be gone. They know that they have low self-esteem, some negative thought pattern, grief, inertia or fear, and they would like nothing more than to be done with it. Most people don't really want to live with pain and suffering, but they just haven't figured out how else to relate to the world.

People want to let go, but they don't always have a method for doing it. How do you let go of a loved one who passes away? How do you let go of an important relationship after a break-up? How do you let events come to a natural conclusion so you can start all over again?

Taoists approach learning meditation in a practical way. They recommend doing what's easy first and leaving what's hard for later on. Build on easy successes before you start trying to take on challenges that may seem impossible. Slowly let your system build up and your internal infrastructure become solid.

The Dissolving method has been used by Taoists for millennia to deal with shock—no matter how serious. The Dissolving method can help you get through incredibly life-altering events. The Dissolving method can help you let go. The actual term in Taoism is *sung shin,* which means "to relax into your heart or being." Here Taoists are talking about the core of your being, about how you connect with your soul.

There are three main applications of the Dissolving method. The first is attending to the here and now. You are basically trying to dissolve blockages that deal with events from your past or your future, but this application is more about what you are aware of at this moment. Whether it comes from your past or not, all energy inside you is going to link together at some point.

The second application of the Dissolving method makes use of agendas. You have something you know you want to do—maybe you have a problem with a relationship, with some aspect of yourself or some aspect of your life's circumstances. In Taoism there is what is classically called the "10,000 agendas." Ten thousand is used as a metaphor for an infinite number of possibilities. You know there are aspects of your life that require change and you want to address each one, individually, as a means of becoming free and awake.

The third application of the Dissolving method helps people to deal with shock. Trauma causes many changes to occur in your system because, by definition, shocking events affect you so deeply. That is, they connect to other blockages and root deeply inside you. Traumas—such as the stock market crash of 1929, September 11, 2001, Hurricane Katrina and the 2008 banking crisis—cause people an incredible amount of shock. If the energy of the shock is not dissolved, it may grow immensely and attach to other blockages, making it increasingly more difficult to release. So you use the technique of dissolving to help release all that has attached to that trauma within you to eventually unravel it to its core.

Regardless of the application, dissolving is a pragmatic method for releasing whatever prevents you from experiencing the joys and harmony inherent in life. Learning these techniques will give you powerful tools for recognizing what is not flowing, releasing it and eventually restoring balance in your life.

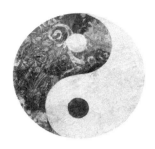

CHAPTER 2
Breathing and Body Awareness

Many forms of meditation can easily become purely cerebral exercises. You are thinking about something, focusing on the middle of your head, and the exercise becomes incredibly brain-centered. In contrast, Taoist meditation incorporates breathing techniques, which serve the very practical function of enabling you to become aware of your body. Taoists use breathing as a powerful tool to become aware of their bodies, their thoughts and the progressively more subtle, deeper layers that drive those thoughts in the first place.

The Stress Response

Taoists hold that the energy running your mind also runs your body, but that these two energies operate at slightly different frequencies. The Western model for understanding the mind is primarily based on the premise that specific emotions and psychological states are created by neurotransmitters. If neurotransmitters are released you experience a corresponding emotional or mental state. In this model your brain functions rather like a computer program—if you can inhibit those neurotransmitters from firing, you can also stop the emotion or mental state from manifesting.

In this sense neurotransmitters also affect the way in which you think on a physical basis. A stress cycle, for example, is caused by increasing levels of chemicals such as noradrenalin and cortisol that are meant to help you in survival situations. Repeated stimulation, however, will slowly but surely downgrade the functions of your body and possibly go so far as to cause a legion of diseases.

Conversely, if you calm down your body, these neurotransmitters will not be triggered. The same goes for the mind. If you calm down both the mind and the body, neither activates a stress response. If you don't, however, either can activate the stress response, creating a negative feedback loop. Medical research claims that meditation is physiologically beneficial and that it benefits both the body and the mind. Meditation provides the method for interrupting the negative feedback loop between body and mind stress.

Longevity Breathing

Taoist whole-body breathing[1] increases your body's ability to effectively use oxygen 24 hours a day. Deep breathing lowers blood pressure, calms unnecessary anxieties and reduces stress and pain by giving your nerves a way to discharge accumulated tension. Breathing well improves the functioning of your body and energy centers; it also clears the mind while balancing the emotions.

The human body has two regular metronomes. One is breath—it goes in and it goes out. If you think that's not really important, try not doing it for a couple of hours. Stop breathing and you'll die. The second rhythm, which is very significant in Taoist meditation, is blood flow. Practicing qigong[2] will give you the ability to control your blood flow and, eventually, the energy flow, or chi, inside your body. Although basic to Taoist training, controlling blood and chi flow is quite difficult to learn because you have to stay present. Working with breathing is easier and serves as a means to access and maintain your awareness.

---

[1] Longevity Breathing is the system the author has developed to teach Taoist whole-body breathing techniques.

[2] Tai chi is a form of qigong. See the author's books *Opening the Energy Gates of Your Body* and *Dragon and Tiger Medical Qigong* to learn more about qigong practices.

There's a wonderful phrase in the Bible, "God formed the man from the dust of the ground and breathed into his nostrils the breath of life, and the man became a living spirit."[3] *Spirit* refers to the Hebrew or Aramaic word meaning breath, energy or soul. You can use your breath as a doorway to your soul or spirit, as a direct link to the depths of your mind, forming a bridge from your conscious to your unconscious mind so you can begin to feel what's stirring underneath. That which is unconscious can drive people crazy and make them spiritually unhealthy rather than spiritually clear.

 ## Personal Practice Session 1

Right now just try to take a good inhale and exhale while putting your attention on your hand. After a couple of breaths, see if you can breathe in and out of your hand. Can you get a feeling of whether oxygen is actually going in and out of your hand? Maybe you can feel something happening. Now try it a few more places. Take a nice deep inhale and see if you can breathe into your forehead. Notice that when you put your attention into your forehead as you breathe, your awareness suddenly expands. You become aware of more subtle feelings than if you were merely thinking about your forehead. Putting your awareness on a specific place in the body amplifies your physiology and the subtle energies inside you.

Now put your attention on your heart. Just try to have the sense that you are breathing in and out of your heart and see if your awareness expands.

 ## Author-guided Practice Session 1

Improve your breathing and awareness: see p. 167.

---

3 Genesis 2:7

Becoming Present

When we can be fully present to our experiences, we see life as it is without filters, and we don't make excuses about why things should or shouldn't be different. We acknowledge the situation we find ourselves in and accept it. With acceptance of life as it is, we gain something else simultaneously—the ability to change. As long as we reject any situation in which we find ourselves, we lose the ability to adapt. Eventually, if we can stay present long enough, we arrive at a point of neither accepting nor rejecting anything, and we can let everything just be.

> *With acceptance of life as it is, we gain something else simultaneously—the ability to change.*

Being present in your life is not determined by where you've been, where you are or where you're going. The excuse that people can't be present because they want something else is not true. You don't find most people running around screaming, "Oh my God, the sun has risen! I really want it to be night. I want the moon!" Taoist practices teach you to become aware of four conditions, which will be discussed in Chapter 4, that signal whether your energy is blocked. When your energy is not blocked, you will simply be present. The degree to which your energy is blocked—for whatever reason—is the degree to which you are incapable of being present.

In addition to all their wonderful health benefits, Longevity Breathing methods give you a way of staying present—a fundamental of Taoist meditation. Breathing is a great tool to help you stay present because your body is always doing it. You can use your breath any time to bring yourself back to the present, especially when you find yourself in any sort of a pickle.

Physiology of the Breath

Doctors report that 90 percent of the American public does not know how to breathe well. Most people do not see the value in breath training because they figure they would be dead if they weren't doing it sufficiently. Yet if you ask them to take a deep breath, they tend to just puff out their chest. I've watched this go on in more than three decades of teaching meditation. Puffing up your chest will not push and pull air in and out of your lungs. It is the diaphragm that moves the air. If you feel down your ribcage and come to the end of the bones, you'll feel something bounce in and out on both sides. That's your diaphragm, and it actually extends all the way to your back. Most of your organs are attached to your diaphragm: liver, spleen, kidneys, glands and digestive valves. Intrinsic to breathing is moving your internal organs, which are meant to have a certain range of motion. Breathing is one of the best ways to keep the organs moving. As your diaphragm loses its range of motion from poor breathing, it affects your health, especially as you age.

The Internal Organs of the Body

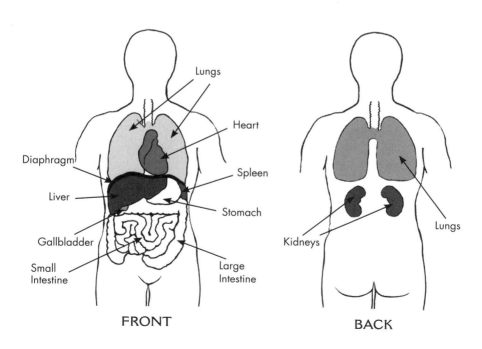

FRONT

BACK

If you let the bottom of your belly go in and out as you breathe, your diaphragm naturally moves down in response to the anatomical connections. When your diaphragm goes down, your lungs fill with air because they are like a big bag with the diaphragm positioned at the bottom. So, let the bag go down and there's space for the air to rush in. When your diaphragm goes up it pushes the air out, expelling carbon dioxide.

 ## Personal Practice Session 2

Place your hands on your belly and breathe in. Don't worry about how much your belly moves—just make sure there is some movement. See if you can get a sense of the breath going down towards the bottom of your belly. When you let go, try to sense your diaphragm rising up and your belly coming back in. Allow your belly to get bigger and smaller with a little upward and downward movement as you inhale and exhale respectively. When you breathe in, have a sense of your diaphragm moving down as your belly expands outward. As you breathe out, have a sense of your diaphragm moving up towards your stomach. Just let the air come in and out, and take your time.

Greatest Transformative Benefit with the Least Effort

To meditate you must learn how to breathe well. The major point of breathing practice in meditation is not for health reasons, but rather to increase your awareness. However, whole-body breath training will help you relax and enjoy wonderful health benefits such as better sleep, reduced stress, greater relaxation and more fulfilling sex.

The autonomic nervous system maintains homeostasis in the body. The sympathetic nervous system, a branch of the autonomic nervous system that is always active at some level, becomes more active during times of stress by controlling the fight-or-flight response. The parasympathetic nervous system is another branch that sends messages to muscle and glandular tissues, either stimulating or inhibiting muscle contraction and glandular secretion. Accordingly, a sympathetic response is generally paired with your inhale and an inhibitory parasympathetic response is paired with your exhale. The relaxation response is naturally connected to exhaling, so havinga good exhale is part of relaxing your system and a great antidote to stress.

If I could only teach one exercise that would have the greatest transformational benefit for the least effort, it would be how to breathe, on a daily basis, with the same full-body, relaxed engagement of a baby. Longevity Breathing techniques are great for everyday life.

From the point of view of Chinese medicine, your internal organs are directly related to your emotions. That is, your emotions function through your internal organs. So the first step towards resolving any emotion starts with becoming present to your experience. You can't drive a car if you don't pay attention to the road. You have to be present to some degree when you cook food or you might burn your house down. Becoming present is essential. Most training in life is about how to be present to the external world. There are incredible universities and educational systems to train your intellect, but not to train your inner world. The inside of you determines the real, day to day quality and wisdom of your life.

 ## Author-guided Practice Session 2

Breathe and move your diaphragm: see p. 167.

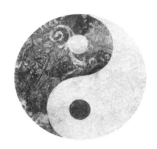

CHAPTER 3
Body Alignments for Sitting Meditation

I f you want to meditate for long periods, you need to learn how to sit well. You want to sit so that your body is in alignment, allowing energy to flow unobstructed. Not sitting well can create various distortions and cause you to focus on all sorts of things that have nothing to do with the task at hand. You may interpret the dull pain from your posture as an emotional issue when in reality it has more to do with your body positioning. For example, your spine might be twisted, causing the energy to move through your acupuncture channels in an awkward way. Habitually incorrect body alignments, such as a twisted spine, may cause a variety of physical or psychological problems including headaches, generalized discomfort and tense thoughts.

Physical Mechanics

The problem of pain brought about by prolonged sitting in a chair, whether in meditation or working at a desk, is caused by the progressive contraction and shortening of the deep muscles and fascia from the bottom of the pelvis to the navel. If this contraction of the thighs, hips and belly is strong enough, the strain will extend higher, and all the soft tissue between your head and your pelvis will be pulled downward. The longer you sit, the more the contraction originating in your pelvis will tighten, fatiguing the muscles, tendons and vertebrae all the way up to your neck and shoulders. Any muscle, tendon or vertebra along the way can easily become misaligned. Contraction in your muscles, in turn, can overstretch your ligaments, stressing your hip and knee joints, causing pain.

The solution lies in stretching out the deep muscles and soft tissue (the ligaments, tendons and fasciae from your knee to the fold between your torso and legs to the lower belly) any time they begin to shorten or fatigue. You accomplish this stretching by making small movements of your pelvis and trunk during sitting. These movements reestablish the nerve signals to the offending muscles, instructing them to keep stretched and not collapse, thus preventing pain and fatigue.

Find Your Alignments

What does it mean to be aligned? An alignment involves two connecting pieces. However, it's not only about connecting, but also about maintaining a smooth flow between the two parts. Each supports the other. When you sit, you start by aligning your body. As you maintain your physical alignments, you eventually learn how to align your energy. This is the second key to proper preparation for meditation.

Whether you sit on the floor[1] or in a chair, make sure your bottom is squarely on the chair. Don't tilt one way or the other. Just let your bottom sit on the chair until it stabilizes and you can let the bones relax. If the floor is too hard, sit on something softer. If you are sitting in a chair, make sure your feet are on the floor; you want to feel your feet aligning with the ground, as if they are connected to it. You also want to have the sense that your legs are growing out of your body, and that your hips and legs feel stable and at ease. You don't want any dissonance. Your legs should feel like two pipes that fit together so that water could flow through them without leaking.

---

[1] Alignments for sitting on the floor are discussed in detail in the author's book, *The Great Stillness*.

Next, check that you have the sense of straightening your spine. Most people, when they sit for long periods, collapse to the left or to the right, but you want to remain positioned in the center, as if a flexible straight beam were running through the middle of you.

If you put your hands on your sides, you will feel something soft between your hips and your ribs—your midriff, or external oblique muscles (see pp. 44–45). Every once in a while you can gently rock from one side to other to open up this area, which is one of the more common contractions—the shrinking in the middle of the body. Then slowly go back to the center. Have the sense of a line dropping from the center of your head right through your pelvis and out of your perineum—the spot between your anus and your genitals at the bottom of your pelvis. If you do this, your back will be straight and you won't lean forward or backward. You should have the sense that the crown of your head is sitting directly over your pelvis.

Go back to your midriff and make sure that you are lifting that area a little. If you have some space there, your diaphragm will not collapse and you'll be able to keep the middle section of your spine fairly straight. Relax your chest and breathe deeply from your belly.

Many people find that their necks are not in the best of shape, so they have to bend their head forward a little. The rule in meditation is that as long as it's stretching your whole spine, you can let your head go forward slightly, but never backward. When you go backward, it shuts down the place between the bottom of your skull and the first vertebra. This scrambles signals coming from your brain down your spine, which can cause feelings of stress and unpleasant sensations in your nerves. If you tilt your head forward, make sure your windpipe isn't constricted. Stay well back from that point. Keep your chin comfortable and relaxed by adjusting your head over your chest and pelvis.

In America, the single most common chiropractic adjustment is between the bottom of the skull and the top of the neck at the atlas axis, or the occipital junction. For various reasons, many people tend to bend their head the wrong way and jam their neck. Open up the very back of your neck just a little so that you feel the top of your neck where it connects to your head. In old Victorian England, if a lady came by, a gentleman would lift his hat ever so slightly off his head. In the same way you want to feel that your skull is raised off your neck very slightly.

Sitting Alignments and Hand Positions

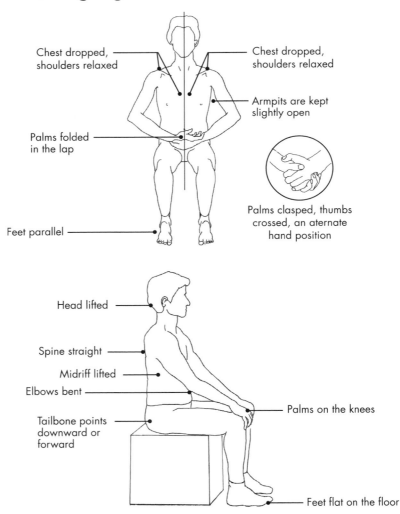

Chest dropped, shoulders relaxed

Chest dropped, shoulders relaxed

Armpits are kept slightly open

Palms folded in the lap

Palms clasped, thumbs crossed, an aternate hand position

Feet parallel

Head lifted

Spine straight

Midriff lifted

Elbows bent

Palms on the knees

Tailbone points downward or forward

Feet flat on the floor

There are three possible positions for your hands. First, you can put them on your thighs close to your knees, keeping the elbows bent. Second, you can fold your hands, one on top of the other, on your lap. It doesn't matter which hand is on top. Most people find the first position easier. You could also fold your hands in your lap so the center of each palm is touching the other. The main point is to make sure your arms are comfortable and don't pull on your spine.

Incorrect Sitting Alignments

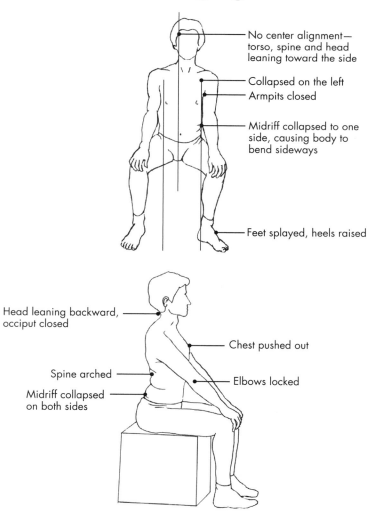

No center alignment— torso, spine and head leaning toward the side

Collapsed on the left
Armpits closed

Midriff collapsed to one side, causing body to bend sideways

Feet splayed, heels raised

Head leaning backward, occiput closed

Chest pushed out

Spine arched

Elbows locked

Midriff collapsed on both sides

Deep Muscles of the Kwa

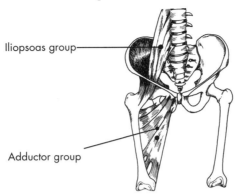

Iliopsoas group

Adductor group

Know Thy Kwa

The part of the body known in Chinese as the *kwa* extends from the inguinal ligament through the inside of the pelvis to the top of the hip bone (one on each side as shown on p. 71).

The trick is to maintain the spring of the soft tissues inside the kwa (see figure above), by eliminating slack or involuntary contractions yet avoiding becoming too taut. To understand this mechanism more fully, think of these muscles and other soft tissues inside your body as a series of interconnected rubber bands. During any period of prolonged sitting—whether in meditation, recreation or office work— you want to maintain the even, continuous tension that allows the rubber bands to exert maximum elasticity and strength. It is the function of the soft tissue to support your body, not the function of the bones, as most people think.

These rubber bands, which bear the weight of your body, are connected to each other. If one of them becomes overly slack, it causes another to become overly taut, pulling in turn on a third. For example, if the pull between the knees and back is excessive, other muscles can overstretch and pull out tendons, ligaments and vertebrae; also, your knee and hip sockets can become misaligned. To understand how your muscles, soft tissues and joints interact as you sit, imagine your soft tissue as a cloth. A length of fabric can be even and smooth or it can have creases. If your body tissues are like smooth cloth, you normally will not experience physical pain or unnecessary fatigue. Creases, however, will ordinarily bring pain and long-term chronic damage, especially when they snap open and close shut again at odd angles. If the cloth is allowed too much slack, it will crumple and crease. If pulled too tight, it may tear somewhere. In the body, cartilage, muscle or ligaments might tear, for example.

Now consider the one continuous piece of cloth as consisting of a spectrum of three colors seamlessly sewn together. The first color band runs from your knee to the inguinal fold at your hip. The second band is what we have identified as the kwa. The kwa regulates the energy in the left and right energy channels of the body. As you can see in the figure, the kwa contains the iliopsoas muscles. One branch begins from the inguinal cut and the floor of the pelvis and continues up to the top of the hip bones, deep inside the pelvis. The other branch is from the thigh bone (femur) to the lower spine. If the soft tissues of the kwa are pulled more than necessary, they negatively affect the lower back and hips. The third color band comprises the deep muscles of the midriff, the internal obliques (located between the crest of the hip bones and the bottom of the ribs) and the continuation of the iliopsoas muscle to the diaphragm.

Each color band affects the other. You need to be aware of each independently, as well as in relation to each other. Let's say the un-creased cloth is 20 inches long, with its top and bottom fixed in space. If you made a crease of 1 or 2 inches in the middle of the cloth, you could cause another part of the cloth to be on the verge of tearing or actually tear, resulting in chronic injury to your knees or hips. If the cloth is not held fixed in space and instead just sags, it can cause the vertebrae to compress and put pressure on nerves inside the body, resulting in both pain and fatigue. When you hit the fatigue point, you have several choices: live with the pain, which can be anything from distracting to physically incapacitating, or restretch your body to its natural length, as if you were removing the creases from the cloth.

The Solution: Stretch and Keep the Kwa Open

The figures below illustrate how the pelvis stretches upward when the kwa opens and collapses when the kwa closes. Opening the kwa is like taking the creases out of the cloth, and closing it is like bringing the creases back. Check that your kwa is open when you begin sitting, and make a special point of checking this at regular intervals. To open your kwa, lift everything you can feel, from your perineum through your pelvis to the top of your hip bones, and then continue feeling a lift through your midriff to the bottom of your ribs, all without lifting your chest. When you accomplish this opening maneuver, the inguinal fold between the top of your leg and the top of your pelvis will straighten (that is, its crease will flatten), relieving pain and reducing fatigue. The opposite happens if your kwa closes and its fold increases—you experience pain and fatigue.

Lifting the Kwa

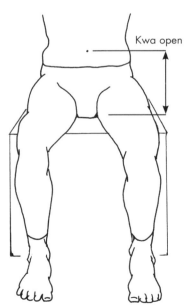
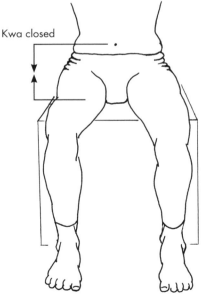

Kwa open   Kwa closed

Correct position;
the kwa is open and lifted.

Incorrect position;
the kwa is closed down.

The kwa must be lifted gently, and not forced, which places the most powerful pressure on your body's "length of cloth." Make sure this gentle lift slowly stretches the soft tissue to your knees and shoulders, so that neither feels pulled or painful. Also, do not deliberately contract your anus as you lift the kwa. The anus will be lifted effortlessly, naturally bringing energy up your body by the kwa action itself.

Exercises to Stretch the Kwa

To alleviate the discomfort of prolonged sitting most people move their shoulders, which does little to help the lower back. The following two exercises not only help the lower back, but also release painful pressure on your shoulders. When the kwa begins to weaken or close, you have two ways to effectively return the body to an uncreased state.

The following suggestions will help you achieve the ideal posture to maintain throughout your sitting meditation:

Gently press the soles of your feet continuously into the ground throughout each exercise to obtain a solid connection from your feet to your spine. Press until your knees feel quite stable, with no slipping or wobbling.

Extend and elongate your muscles upward from your knees to and through your kwa, all the way up to your lowest ribs. If done well, this stretching will noticeably release the muscles of your lower, middle and upper back as well as your shoulders and neck—without deliberately moving them. Depending on your size and the original amount of contraction in your kwa, your body could lengthen anywhere from half an inch to 3 inches. The better you become at mentally relinquishing the contraction of your nerves, the bigger the stretch and release of the torso.

You can use both exercises when you feel your body beginning the slippery slide to ever-worsening contraction or when you feel your mind weakening and becoming distracted. Begin with the simple external movements offered in Exercises 1 and 2. Both are performed in the same way and yield the same benefits when meditating in a chair or on the floor. Your hands should remain in your choice of one of the three previous palm positions described on p. 44.

Exercise 1: Moving the Spine Forward and Backward and in Circles

1. Continuously keep your spine absolutely straight—without hunching your back—from your tailbone to the top of your head.

2. Bend forward from your inguinal fold and return to your original starting point slowly and rhythmically so that you gradually re-stretch your kwa and midriff. The bend will usually be in the range of 3 to 18 inches. Use the 70 percent rule as a guideline to know how far to stretch forward without exceeding your limits. If you are meditating, bend only as far as you need to both comfortably maintain your internal work and relieve your body of distracting pain. If you use this exercise to relieve the pain from desk work at the office, you may want to pause for a moment and put your full attention on rehabilitating your back. Your increased productivity will more than compensate for the time lost. Remember, this movement is in the long-term interest of your back. The Dalai Lama even does a few-inch version of this excercise during his teachings.

3. Maintaining the straight spine described in step 1, stretch your kwa and midriff by moving your body in a circle. First lean your whole spine slightly forward, to the right, slightly back, to the left and forward again, using the center of your pelvis as the center of your circle. As you execute this circling, it is important to extend continuously from your perineum through the center of your body, up the front of your spine and out from the top of your head. Pay particular attention to stretching from the knee through the kwa and midriff when you get to the left and right sides of the circle. Do your best to even out any imbalance on either side by moving more slowly or extending higher on the more contracted side. Pay extra attention to lifting the kwa when moving

through the sides of the circle. The Dalai Lama and many Tibetan Buddhist Rinpoches also use this method although they only move side-to-side, not in circles.

Next, repeating all three steps, make a second circle, moving your body in the opposite direction to balance your small internal stretches.

Exercise 2: The Sitting Spine Stretch

1. Bend your spine slightly forward by focusing on releasing the back of your vertebrae, one by one, beginning from your tailbone and progressively moving upward to the top of your neck (A–D).

The Sitting Spine Stretch, First Half

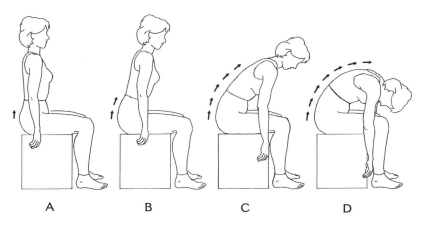

A   B   C   D

A: Starting posture. The back is straight, head lifted, chest dropped, belly relaxed and shoulders rounded.

B–D: Gradually release the vertebrae from bottom to top, bending forward with each release. Release from the back of the vertebrae.

2. Raise the vertebrae of your spine by focusing on pushing up from deep inside your belly and the front of your vertebrae, one by one, again beginning from your tailbone and moving to the top of your head (E–H).

3. If one side of your body is more contracted than the other, emphasize pushing up the kwa on the side that is near the contraction. In other words, if your left side is more contracted, apply more effort for the kwa on the left side than for the kwa on the right side.

The Sitting Spine Stretch, Second Half

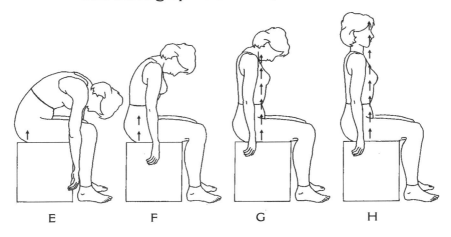

E   F   G   H

E: Posture upon completion of first half (you are bent all the way forward).

F–H: As you sit up straight, open[2] the front of the spine from bottom to top.

---

2 "Open" means lifting each vertebra in the front (vertebrae are already opened in back from the first part of the stretch).

Two advanced techniques, kwa pulsing and pumping the spinal fluid, are also important to sitting meditation but are beyond the scope of this book.[3] The internal work necessary to do both techniques is taught as part of my core qigong program, which also encompasses the sixteen components of Taoist neigong.

 ## Author-guided Practice Session 3

Find your alignments more easily and get help maintaining them: see p. 167.

Sit Well, Be Grounded

Be present to your body when sitting. Lean a little forward and then go back a little until you find the balance point where a straight line is created down the very middle of your body, in front of your spine and behind your chest, belly and hips. Once you can maintain it, scan down from the top of your head, feel whether your body is aligned and adjust as necessary. Sit well. Be grounded.

Let this be a metaphor about being aligned with other things in your life. Is the work you do to eat your daily bread aligned with what you feel you should be doing in this life? Are you doing crazy things for crazy reasons? Can you recognize it? If you are behaving in ways that others might find crazy but the reasons make sense to you, then whether your actions are "crazy" is, frankly speaking, an opinion. But, if your actions seem crazy to you, yet you continue doing them to satisfy somebody or something somewhere else, consider whether your life is really aligned. Is the way you live your life, where you live, how you live, aligned with where you would like to go in life? If not, you probably will never reach your desired destination.

If your head is not sitting correctly on your shoulders it could mean that your job is not really right for you. Sitting with your midriff lifted, your spine straight and your head over your pelvis might, one day,

---

[3] See the author's book, *Opening the Energy Gates of Your Body*, pp. 163–165 and 40 respectively.

make you see into relationships you have with people and look at how well they are aligned. Sitting is a method for recognizing what is flowing and what is blocked. Inner wisdom often comes in the simplest of ways. Many ordinary activities are metaphors for everything else in life. Sitting is one of them.

When you sit, do you have the sense that you are grounded? Is there something inside you that's very stable while you sit? This grounding doesn't only come from your body, but it also includes an internal feeling of stability. This is the place from which you want to begin any sort of meditation practice. It's the place you want to be if you genuinely want to pray or engage in any form of spirituality. Finding this point allows everything to integrate.

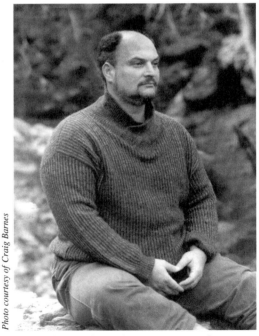

Photo courtesy of Craig Barnes

The author is shown here practicing the Inner Dissolving method.

Does your chest feel as though it's resting above your belly comfortably? As you lift your midriff does your diaphragm move freely and easily? Let the pressurization in your chest go through your diaphragm and transfer to your internal organs (see pp.36–38), so the top of your body is connected and aligned with the bottom of your body. As your body becomes unified, your mind and spirit become one whole cloth, instead of fabric torn in many places.

As you move down to your pelvis, notice if your head connects with it. Do you need to raise your head or spine? Is everything aligned from the bottom of your pelvis, up to the top of your head and your arms? Does your body feel like one piece or a bunch of disconnected parts? See if you can link the pieces.

Let your hands connect down through your legs to your feet. Are they aligned and connected to the rest of your body? One body aligned can become one mind, one spirit. By being in a stable sitting position you allow your awareness to naturally expand and keep the energy channels open. Chi is then free to flow, making it much easier to let go of any blockages you've been holding. Having your body aligned, centering in your belly—the exact center of your body, with as much above it as below it—creates a natural stability point. From that stability point, it becomes much easier to meditate.

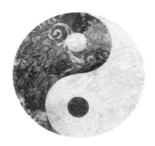

CHAPTER 4
Blockages: Recognizing the Four Conditions

The Water method of Taoist meditation says that if you take away all that is false, all you will be left with is that which is true. According to the Water tradition, challenges such as injury, illness and emotional or physical issues are characterized by blockages.

All blockages can be identified in one of four ways:

- Strength

- Tension

- Something that doesn't feel quite right, even if you don't know what it is

- Any kind of contraction.

As you start the Dissolving process at the top of your head, scan downwards and note whether you find one or more of the four conditions present in your body.

Strength

Everybody wants to be strong. Have you ever met anybody who's selling a weakness pill? Nobody would really like to be completely weak, impotent and useless in the world. So in the West there is a lot of emphasis on strength. In meditation, however, strength has a completely different meaning.

Taoists don't typically use the word *ego*, but there's a kind of strength that produces an ego. It's the voice that says, "This is what I will do: I will make the world be the way I want it to, no matter what obstacles must be overcome." This creates a lot of pressure and stress. Strength can be stubbornness, which leaves you with the inability to change. When you are too stubborn, you feel strong. Strength can also be connected to anger. Who doesn't feel strong when they get angry?

The Taoists say that when you really *have it,* you don't notice it. What this means is that generally, when everything is working well, you aren't aware of it and you don't have a feeling of strength. You just feel at ease and natural. When your energy is flowing smoothly, you don't feel strong; you feel comfortable. When you feel strength, it's usually because you are relentlessly pushing and straining. Eventually you snap. Take the classic Type-A personality who is highly successful but suddenly drops dead from a heart attack caused by overwork.

Do you have high blood pressure? If you train yourself to become more sensitive, you can feel when your blood is forcing its way through your system. Likewise, when people get incredibly fixated on their thoughts and ideas—on what they believe and think is true—they are acting from strength. Everything then becomes rigid rather than flexible. You want to be able to recognize when you're feeling a blockage of strength. Where are you trying too hard in your life? Where are you forcing your body too much? In what life circumstances are you finding yourself continuously frustrated, angry or overwhelmed?

Personal Practice Session 3

Start at the top of your head, close your eyes and sit up straight. Become present to the fact that you are sitting in a chair or on the floor. What does your body feel like when it sits? What does the chair or floor feel like? Slowly scan down your body inch by inch and notice if you feel any strength. It may be very subtle or it can be very obvious from the beginning. Can you relax that strength? Can you be present to it? You don't have to push. You can just let it be there. Gradually it will reduce of its own accord.

Move down to your forehead, down to your eyes, where a lot of tension and strength accumulates. Staring at computer screens can lead to feelings of strength from the repeated flipping between windows and seeking data in seconds before going to the next screen. The physical memory—the flashes, bits and bytes—stay locked in the eyes and optic nerve unless we relax and stop the eyes from going out. When you feel strength in your eyes, notice what thoughts are behind those images, behind your eyes.

Move down your face to your mouth. Notice and become aware. Move down to your throat. Are you exerting more strength in your voice than is necessary? Move down your chest. Is there strength in your heart? Is your heart soft enough that you can actually listen to what is deeper inside you?

Down into your belly where your internal organs are, do you feel strength there? Forget about six-pack abs (whether you have them or not), the blubber on your belly or the size of your stomach. What is underneath those abdominals, those muscles that you can see? It's your internal organs—they keep you healthy or become diseased. Do you feel strength in your internal organs? Do they feel tight or clogged up? What do your guts feel like? Do you feel strength or are they soft and smooth?

As you move from the top of your head to the bottom of your belly, keep noticing if you are holding any strength in your body. Recognize it. Be present to what's happening and how you feel. Don't stop anything from happening— just let it flow as if you were floating down a river. Think of your thoughts, emotions and body as leaves that fall into a river and drift away downstream.

Tension

The second of the four conditions indicating blocked energy is tension. Tension always involves a fight. Something is seeking dominance over something else. It could be something as small as how you are going to make a deadline—how you are going to accomplish the task versus the amount of time you have to do it. Being angry is an example of emotional tension. Someone or something has broken a boundary and you want to it to remain intact. Two things are pulling in opposite directions. Being angry is a more yang emotion, but depression is just as powerful as anger. It is a more inward or yin type of emotional tension. Can you recognize if you have any tension inside you from other emotions like greed or grief?

What causes tension and pulls you in opposite directions in your life? You are here, but you want to be there. Should you be with this person or that person? You are ready, but the opportunity hasn't presented itself. Don't overlook the fights that might be occurring inside your body. Maybe your tissues are constantly tense—knots pull your muscles in opposite directions.

Personal Practice Session 4

Sit straight so your body is not collapsed. Start at the top of your head and notice if you can find any tension in your body. Tension of thought is not exactly the same as tension in the body. High blood pressure is not the same as tension of thought. A tense thought can pass fairly easily, whereas high blood pressure takes a little more effort to bring down. Tense thoughts, however, can create high blood pressure quite easily. Terrify people until they think they're going to die or experience some sort of violent situation and their heartbeat suddenly goes up to 170 or even 210 beats per minute. They can't see; their vision narrows almost to a pinpoint and they lose peripheral vision. Muscles that worked fine minutes before are paralyzed. It's all the result of high stress levels. You get similar although less extreme reactions with lower stress levels. So this is tension.

Start by closing your eyes so you can focus your attention inwardly. More advanced Taoist meditation is done with the eyes open, but it's not done that way in the beginning because what you see outside might distract you. You are taking an inward journey to recognize what is inside of you. Again, you'll start at the top and feel the crown of your head. Do you have any tension there? If you pay attention and don't let yourself do anything but notice, becoming aware of feelings and sensations, in most cases tension in your head will present itself, even if it is very subtle. So be aware of the reality of your experience whether you think it should be happening or not.

Scan down your head to your forehead. You are recognizing your body and becoming aware of any tension. Maybe a thought will come into your head. Don't pay much attention to the thought itself, but instead notice if it's a tense thought. Happy thoughts are usually relaxed while tense thoughts usually pit you against the "other."

As you scan your body, can you feel the tension in a thought that leads to an emotion? We all know what it feels like to be excited, to feel optimistic and to have a good time. We all know what it feels like to be angry, sad or disappointed. Emotions create subtle body feelings. Usually they're not gross, but they're there. This explains why people can stuff their anxiety all day long and implode in the evenings after work. All of a sudden what was subtle turns into a generalized mood, which can eventually become a very strong emotion. Notice the emotional energy you feel inside your body. Do you have tense emotions of anger, sadness or fear that need to be released? What does it feel like to be happy, content and at peace with yourself?

Continue down inch by inch to your jaw. Most people carry a lot of tension in their jaw. Many habitually grind their teeth in their sleep to the point of wearing down their molars. So what is that tension? What is in your jaw? Become aware of the reality of the situation. Don't try to change it; don't do anything with it. You are only observing what's there. Next, go down to your shoulders and, again, become present to any tension. Tension and strength are related, but tension always involves a fight, affecting thoughts, emotions, your body and the energy that runs through you. As you become able to observe progressively more subtle layers, you will discover deeper levels of tension. There's no magic here, just learning to pay close attention to the reality of what's occurring.

Move down to your chest and pay particular attention when you reach your heart. In the West, the fast pace of modern life has made heart disease one of today's leading causes of death. Continue down a bit farther to your belly. Can you distinguish between the upper and lower parts of your belly, going down an inch or two below your belly button? As your mind seems to naturally come to a stop, become aware of the tension inside of you. What is holding you back? See if it will relieve itself before rushing to continue.

Be aware of how paying attention to your tension can make you want to run away or go to sleep and avoid it. People avoid that which is unpleasant; and when they finally do focus on something unpleasant, they often push it down. Then it can come back with a vengeance, perhaps in a different form or place. So just be aware of what's inside you. You can continue this practice for as long as you'd like as often as you like.

When Something Doesn't Feel Quite Right

The third of the four conditions is tricky. Our inner worlds are filled with an amazing amount of congestion. Most people are not even aware of what's there. As infants, we have many experiences before we understand and can use language. When we were in our mother's womb, we picked up everything that happened to our mother. If she was yelled at, if she was beaten, if she underwent stress, if she drank, if people around her were putting out incredibly negative vibes that she was soaking up—any of these situations disturbed us. Conversely, if she was incredibly happy, content and peaceful, we picked that up too.

There are a million connections between dendrites in the brain. Experiences get wired with a cornucopia of input. All you know is that something doesn't feel right. It is one thing to know what bothers you, but quite another when you haven't got the faintest clue. You may never get to the bottom of it, but something that doesn't feel quite right will become a part of your real, ongoing experience. When people can't figure out what is bothering them, they get frustrated or feel helpless—and that may lead to lashing out, running away or getting depressed. So you must be present to these feelings even if you can't seem to identify where they are coming from. These feelings account for the malaise and confusion in the world. Some people appear to have everything anyone could

> *Some people appear to have everything anyone could ever want yet life doesn't seem to flow for them.*

ever want yet life just doesn't seem to flow for them. You have to be present to what you are feeling. When you become present, you can apply your intent to get rid of what holds you back using the Dissolving method, which the next chapter discusses in detail.

People have incredible memories locked deep inside their systems from birth. One man, whose mother had been in labor 52 hours before giving birth to him, had physical hallucinations his entire life as a result. I treated him with qigong tui na[1] to help relieve this condition. We have no words, no understanding and no pictures as we come down that canal in total, absolute blackness, but our brain still registers what we felt about the experience. Many times when people refer to their past-life experiences, they may actually be talking about the birthing process or what happened in their mother's womb.

Later, during your first year as a baby, you don't yet understand language but there are constant sounds and impulses coming at you. The nervous system is extremely fragile, so babies have all kinds of unpleasant experiences. They frequently get diarrhea, painful gas or stomach upsets, and all they know is that they're feeling tortured. They have no idea where the pain is coming from or why. Some people get over this and some people don't. It depends on how intense the experiences were, how much they affected their nervous system and brain, and how resilient their nervous system was at birth. This is one example of why something inside you might not feel quite right, but you don't know what it is.

---

[1] *Qigong tui na* or "energy bodywork" is a sophisticated medical qigong system with 200 hand techniques, which are used for healing. In this specialty of Chinese medicine, the healer directly emits and rebalances the chi in the patient's body to bring about a therapeutic result. Its diagnostic techniques are based on reading the energy of the external aura, as well as the subtle energy of the internal tantiens (similar to chakras) of the body.

In the Far East wealthy families traditionally build a separate cottage when a woman becomes pregnant. Only her relatives are allowed in and they are not allowed to say negative things or cause any problems in her presence. The best possible environment is set up for the mother so that the energy flowing into the child is very peaceful. Sometimes the mother-to-be would be taken to a place where no one else lived within a mile so she couldn't even hear the neighbors fighting.

 ## Personal Practice Session 5

Sit up straight and begin to bring your body into alignment. When your body is bent and crooked, unnecessary physiological distractions will come up. Starting at the top of your head and scanning downward, become present and aware of what doesn't feel quite right, especially if you don't know what it is. Recognize, feel and sense it. Don't feel any pressure to know what this feeling is; just recognizing is enough. When you reach the middle of your forehead, take a little more time on the third eye, between and a little higher than your eyebrows. This is where many people find it easier to become aware of increasingly subtle sensations in their nervous systems. Notice if you find hints of strength, tension or anything that doesn't feel quite right, especially if you do not know what it is or even what it might be. Then move down to your throat.

If you've done the preceding scanning exercises you might find that it's becoming easier for you to stay present now that you have a little experience. Move down to your chest and take as much time as you need before moving down to your belly. Does anything not feel quite right? Forget what you look like on the outside; your reality has more to do with how you are living on the inside. Is your inner life rich or poor? Move all the way down to the bottom of your belly,

an inch or two below your belly button. Is there any strength, ten-
sion, or something that doesn't feel quite right? Be present to any
of these conditions.

Contraction

The fourth condition is contraction. The primary difference between
someone who is very awake and someone who is sleepwalking
through life is that someone who is awake is not contracted. Someone who is closed down or contracted is half asleep.

What people call ego, stress and the fear of living are examples
of contraction. Likewise, blood vessels closing down and organs
malfunctioning are also examples of contractions. Rather than being open and operating fluidly, certain parts of the body start to
contract and eventually shut down. The Taoists call contraction the
"hallmark of death." A thousand diseases can be described as
simply something in the body closing down. For example, a heart
attack results from the interruption of blood supply to the heart when
a coronary artery becomes clogged to the point of shutting down.

 ## Personal Practice Session 6

As you begin scanning downward from the top of your
head, consider this question: What is a contraction? Is any-
thing pulling against something else? Become aware of and
be present to any contraction in the top of your head. How
do you feel it in your body? How do you feel contraction in
your overall sense of yourself? Is something closing down?
Move down to your forehead and notice if there are any
contractions in your skull and brain. Maybe a contraction
exists in one of the plates of your skull. Maybe when you
are feeling sensations in your head, you are actually feeling
a contraction in your brain. Somehow it's casting its shad-
ow as fatigue or indifference. If you are really present, you

will hear everything that is happening—every sound in the room. When your awareness contracts, you can no longer be aware or present to your experience. You shut down.

Move down to your throat, the seat of expression. There are bound to be memories in there of how your speech wasn't as honest, clear and clean as you might have wanted it to be. Nobody is perfect—in fact, nobody is even close. Let go of contractions where you lacked courage or where you just couldn't rise to the challenge. Slowly move toward a more solid foundation where you're not collapsing on yourself structurally, energetically and emotionally, or feeling mentally frustrated and narrow-focused.

Move down to your chest. Long before a heart attack comes on, there may be feelings of tightening in the chest. Most people cannot be present to the experience: They can't feel the subtle changes, they don't recognize them. They may skip medical appointments either to avoid a short-lived unpleasant experience or because they are not even aware that something is wrong. The condition of contraction makes you unable to muster the energy to be proactive.

Move down to your belly, where all the internal organs reside that maintain your life: your liver, spleen, intestines and kidneys (see p. 37). What do they feel like if they become contracted? Most people can't feel their organs, but you can become more sensitive to them as you get a sense of what's going on in your body.

 ## Author-guided Practice Session 4

Dissolve strength, tension, something that doesn't feel quite right or any kind of contraction: see p. 167.

Putting It All Together

Take some time to focus on each of the four conditions separately. Next, focus on strength and tension. When you have stabilized your ability to scan and stay present to strength and tension, move on to see if you can recognize anything that doesn't feel quite right. Eventually you want to put everything together and be present to any of the four types of blockages that call out for your attention.

 ## Personal Practice Session 7

Begin at the top of your head and become present to sensations or experiences of any kind. You understand the process now. Move slowly from the top of your head to the bottom of your belly, becoming aware of any of the four conditions. Move down your body inch by inch, giving equal attention to the front, sides and back. As you descend, imagine that your awareness is a peaceful waterfall covering everything as the water rushes down. You scan your front, side and back at the same time. This is the process of becoming present to what is going on inside you, finding out whether energy is flowing inside you or whether it is blocked.

Fold your hands in front of your stomach, gently resting them where you can feel the rising and falling in coordination with your inhale and exhale. Inhale and let your belly get a little bigger with a sense of downward pressure. Exhale and just relax and let everything go. When your diaphragm reaches all the way to the bottom of its range of motion, you'll naturally feel the exhale begin, so just follow it. Let your breath relax you and exhale without holding your breath. At the end of the exhale, allow the inhale to come back of its own accord. On the next exhale, really let everything go, but don't force it. Then on the inhale, put your attention on any place where you have strength, tension, something that doesn't feel quite right, even if you don't know what it is, or any kind of contraction.

Use your inhale to make you more aware of any of those four conditions. When you exhale, just relax and let everything flow naturally out of them. Breathe in and identify any problem spots. Breathe out and release each one, letting whatever it is resolve.

Start again at the top of your head. Breathe into this area and breathe out. Breathe in and become aware of any of those four conditions. Exhale and let them dissipate. Inhale and notice if you feel strength. Exhale and let it go as best you can. When you inhale, if you feel something and you don't understand what it is, don't try to define it. Just exhale and let go. Let it relax and calm down. When you inhale just recognize if you have a contraction. Exhale and let go. If on the inhale you feel strength, but you haven't quite grasped what it is, exhale and go deeper into it. Inhale from that deeper place and recognize it more fully. Then exhale again. Inhale and exhale several times in that same spot until something that was vague, whether you understand it or not, becomes very tangible to you.

Eventually that which you couldn't feel will become clear. All of a sudden you'll realize, "Oh, that's what it is. This is what I've been feeling all day long without realizing what it's about." Then let go and really relax. Do this a couple of times. Inhale and recognize what's there, then exhale and let go of it.

When you are ready, move down your head a little further to somewhere in your forehead—maybe it's the front or maybe it's the back of your head. Do you feel some tension? Breathe into and out of that place a couple of times until you go from feeling that something is out of your reach to at least being clear that it's there. Again, inhale and exhale to become even more aware of it. Exhale and let it go. Inhale and become more aware. Exhale and let it relax.

When you are ready, go to the next place down in your head where you find some tightness or other sensation—maybe your eyes, a common source of tension for people who stare at computers all day. Try to sit up straight so you don't put yourself into some kind of trance. Breathe into your eyes and then let go. Is it strength? Tension? Something that doesn't feel quite right, even if you don't know what it is? Some kind of contraction? Breathe in and out of this space—one, two, three, four times until it becomes tangible to you, something you can recognize. The four conditions can show themselves in many ways—maybe in your eyes, through a buzz you feel inside your nerves, words that pop up in your head or flickering images that may stir up positive or negative emotions. Whether you fully understand it or not doesn't matter. Exhale a couple of times and let it go.

Move your attention down to the next place in your body where you feel one of the four conditions, possibly somewhere in your chest, heart or throat. Again, see if you can feel what is inside you as you breathe in and out a couple of times. If you notice one of the four conditions, just sit with it and see if you can allow that blockage to amplify a bit. If you breathe a few times, it becomes less subtle and increasingly obvious. When you think you know which condition it is, or at least have some idea, exhale and let go. Again, inhale and become more aware of the blockage. Exhale and let go for a couple of breaths.

As you do this, you develop your ability to recognize any of the four conditions: strength, tension, something that doesn't feel quite right, especially if you don't know what it is, or any kind of contraction. You are developing the ability to stay with a blockage and not get distracted. Use your breath to stay focused. Breathe into your belly. Breathe out of your belly. Gently become aware of any areas that are calling out for your attention. Let go with each exhale and as you breathe in, let the blockage come into focus. Relax it with your exhale. If you can't release the entire blockage, breathe in again and when you exhale, let it go as much as you can. Relax.

Energy Anatomy

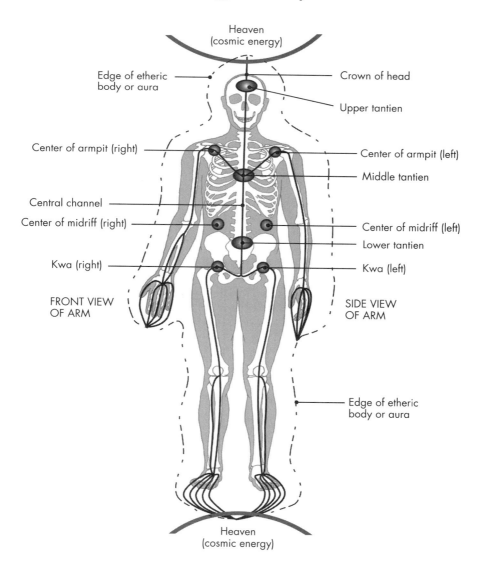

Continue to move down bit by bit, stopping at any place that calls attention to itself. Maybe you have a particular physical problem, or you maybe you discover a place of tension you hadn't noticed before. Breathe into it. You might recognize subliminal tension and stress inside any part of your body where you've had an operation. Breathe into it. Become aware of the stress and tension residing there and exhale to help it go away. Continue breathing into that space until it becomes clearer. As you become more conscious of the blockage, let it go. Continue down to an inch or two below your navel. This is your lower tantien, one of three major centers in the body where chi collects, disperses and recirculates (see figure on p. 71). You are developing the ability to actually feel what's happening inside your inner world. This is the beginning of learning the breathing process. You breathe into the different spots of your body and then you let them go.

The Present Is Freedom

For millennia Taoists have found that recognizing these four conditions enables people to focus on where their energy is blocked. You first must become present, or you will not be able to explore what is not working inside you. All human beings need regular rhythms to integrate their experiences or they simply become overwhelmed. When the water breaks the dam, real problems begin to happen. Whether horrible or good things happen, if you have the ability to be present, you can handle whatever situation arises.

One day when studying in Beijing with my teacher Liu, I made a comment that showed I was missing the point of meditation. I announced, "I would really like to be happy all the time." Certainly people the world over have had the same wish. Liu took one look at me and laughed aloud. He replied, "Would you really like to live in a place where the weather was always perfect, the temperature never changed and every day was exactly the same?" He pointed out that in a short period of time I would not only get bored, but I would also find that the lack of variation in life was taking away all the joy of living.

When you become present and accept life as it is, freedom will come with it. You have the space inside yourself to decide to do something different and then change that direction. When you don't accept life as it is, you become like an addict chasing one high after another. You get stuck and lose your ability to change. It doesn't matter what you do or how you do it, how strong your will might be or how tough or disciplined you are because you are caught in a continuous loop. You will make yourself the hamster on a wheel. You have to integrate your experiences because you can't run or hide from your inner world.

Freedom is about letting go and being open to change. At the end of the day, freedom always involves change. As you release blockages at ever greater levels, you will find that the light inside you begins to shine and you aren't so driven by your own personal agendas. The Taoists always started by establishing this flow in the body. Letting go of physical strength, tension, anything that doesn't feel quite right and any kind of contraction will be amongst your first challenges.

> *Freedom is about letting go and being open to change.*

Make Time Anytime

The first question on people's lips usually has to do with how much or how often to practice. Generally speaking, you want to practice a minimum of three times a week. For the first three years it is strongly recommended to practice for a minimum of 10 to 20 minutes per session at least three or four times a week. Daily is best. Experienced meditators can practice considerably longer than this, some even for many hours a session.

The optimum times to practice may not be realistic for most people. As with most energy development exercises, the best time to practice begins about two hours before dawn, which is when the earth is most quiet and psychic disturbance is lowest. Another good time is early in the morning, around sunrise. It's best to practice on an empty stomach in the morning so that the energy of the body is not dissipated by digesting a meal. Have breakfast afterwards.

If you can't practice in the morning, then practice in the afternoon or at night. You can even practice on your lunch break or anytime you find yourself getting stressed out or under the gun. You'll make up the 15 minutes by letting go of some of the obstacles that will keep tripping you up throughout your day. Forcing and pushing through can only be maintained for so long.

Your ability to progress in any form of meditation depends strongly on your particular karmic makeup and on the kind and quantity of internal obstacles present. Progress in meditation is not linked directly to time spent in practice.

Practicing sometimes is better than not practicing at all; practicing regularly every day is better than practicing irregularly; and practicing twice a day is better than practicing once a day. Taking a few days or weeks alone or in a group at a meditation retreat—away from the distractions of worldly life—is also helpful. Many people need a week or more just to quiet down the external noise so they can become present to what is inside them. Meditation groups have long existed all over the world to help people learn strategies to apply in their daily lives.

When people buy a product or service they have a reasonable right to know what it is going to do and how long it will take to work. But meditation is not a product. However much or little you practice, it only gives you an opportunity to gain access to yourself—it does not give you a guarantee.

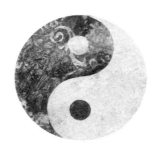

CHAPTER 5
The Dissolving Method:
A Process of Letting Go

We've discussed the four conditions that help you recognize energy blockages in your body. Logically we may know that letting go of obstacles—our inner demons and challenges—is a good idea because the past doesn't exist anymore. But when they exist in your mind, they're very real to you even if they don't actually exist anywhere else. If you talk to someone in their 50s who is still controlled by their parents, even if the parents died 15 years prior, they will respond as if those traumatic events are still happening. The mind holds on and, if you don't make a concerted effort to let go, it will continue recreating experiences inside you in 10,000 different ways. It's bad enough to go through a terrible event once, but it's absolutely horrible to have to continue reliving that experience again and again over 20, 30 or 40 years of your life.

All of us accumulate an incredible amount of clutter in our inner world. We build up mountains of ideas and tension. We very often believe that what we think about is what life is, but we never actually reach what's below the surface. Some of the happiest people on the face of the earth have no education. Some of the most educated people in the world are completely miserable all the time. If you don't let go of what makes you unhappy—at least that which you are aware of—you can expect to keep it for all time.

The Eight Energy Bodies

The Taoists found that human beings encompass eight energy bodies that spiral into the energy of the universe. Chi, your vital life-force energy, flows through each of the energy bodies, which vibrate at increasingly higher frequencies inside you. The eight energy bodies connect you to the energy bodies of all living organisms throughout the universe.

The Eight Energy Bodies:

1. The flesh of the physical body.

2. The chi body, which fuels the physical body.

3. The emotional body, which gives rise to your emotions, both positive and negative.

4. The mental body, which causes thoughts to function, whether with clarity or confusion.

5. The psychic body, which allows us to find our hidden internal capacities and helps our intuition or psychic perceptions become concrete.

6. The causal body, which causes karma to flow.

7. The body of individuality, which enables the actual birth of the full spiritual being commonly referred to as our essence.

8. The realization of the Tao or the entire universe, which few people ever actualize.

These energy fields comprise all the aspects that humans can experience regardless of time, place or circumstances. They are in effect maps that enable you to systematically become aware of the layers of your consciousness and the chi blockages they each hold. Eventually the way your energetic field links you to the energies of other human beings and the universe becomes relevant.

Nervous Tension

In previous eras, physical labor was a huge part of life—people plowed fields and had to do manual labor to earn money for their food and shelter. That's not how most people operate in today's jumpy world. This electronic age is constantly assaulting your nervous system. Most people will tell you they're relaxed when you can visibly see their tension. The computer and almost everything in the modern world makes people tense. Television programs don't even hold the same frame for more than 15 seconds because people lack the attention span for it. Entertainment is one aspect, but, more importantly, we are losing the ability to stay present to what is happening in our own lives.

Most people are unaware that they habitually tense and strain; and, if they are aware, they probably have no idea to what extent. Letting go has to have a certain amount of appeal to you before you can actually start the process. If you don't see a problem in the first place, you're going to have a difficult time trying to fix it. You must recognize that you are constantly straining and tensing. We've been brought up our whole life to seek control—to control what happens now, what happens next. The trouble is that we cannot control the external world. You can become awake, allow it to be, allow it to work and make your accommodations, but the point of meditation is not to learn how to be more in control. Meditation is meant to help you release the need for control in the first place. Every time people have emotional meltdowns, each time they jump and try to hold on to control, they find they can do it for a few minutes, but cannot maintain it. So how do we let go of the need to control what's inside of us?

Letting Go into Happiness

Taoists put a lot of consideration into letting go, which they called *dissolving*. When sugar dissolves in water, the sugar lets go of its separate characteristics and just becomes part of the water. Letting go is the easiest way to describe what people in the ancient world called dissolving.

If you watch a thought long enough, it will just disappear and another one will come along to replace it. Then another will replace that one. That's not what letting go is about. Letting go is going behind what generates every thought, feeling and sensation until you reach the one place where everything attaches to the nexus or the root of the tree. For happiness to well up inside of you, whatever is stopping it has to leave to make room. To hold pain inside you, a terrible memory has to remain intact for you to continuously relive it. Letting go is about releasing whatever stops you from being happy and, equally, keeps you miserable.

Typically, people do not consciously think, "Well, I know I need to let go of this now." They don't recognize the 10,000 connections attached to a given blockage that allows it to continue to exist and progress. In essence, they don't know how to get to the root of the symptoms that blockage is throwing up. Likewise, if and when they subsequently do get rid of the blockage, most of the time they'll never know how it happened. If we're honest, don't we all have a character flaw we wish we would address? We want to get rid of it, but we don't always get to the energy behind that effect to see what's driving it in the beginning.

Whatever you are holding on to, whether it's a demon or an angel, will connect to other blockages inside you. It's unlikely that you are ever going to be able to make sense of these links intellectually. To know what something is, you have to be able to think about it. You couldn't think in the womb. You couldn't think or speak the first few months of your life. So from the perspective of where you sit today, how could you possibly know what it was that got locked inside you at that time? You cannot articulate what you do not know, but those sensations and feelings are still very much there, controlling you from the inside.

In times past, tension in human beings generally involved the muscles and physical body. Today tension comes from the way we use our minds. The more we use our minds, the more skilled the mind becomes at hiding what is deep inside that makes it difficult for us to let go.

The 10,000 ways of being in denial, fooling ourselves, the masks we wear, they all prevent us from understanding what is really going on. Maybe you won't ever realize you are imprisoned. Maybe you won't know if your prison has steel or gold bars. But, if you've ever found yourself in prison, locked behind bars, and you get the chance to open the door and walk out into the sunlight, does it really matter how you got in there and why? The important point is that you get out, that it's finally over. Can you finally let go? Can you finally relax into your spirit? Are you willing to let whatever joy is naturally inside of you come out? Can you finally go from the prison of being half-dead into the light of being fully alive?

> *The more we use our minds, the more skilled the mind becomes at hiding what is deep inside that makes it difficult to let go.*

You have learned how to scan through your entire body from the top of the head down, feeling for every single place where there is strength, tension, something that doesn't feel quite right, especially if you don't know what it is, or any type of contraction. This is the basic Water method Taoists have used for thousands of years to recognize where energy is blocked.

Now that you know what is blocked you need to know how to fix it. If you are fine to leave it inside you for the time being while you work on other blockages or generate the chi you need to deal with it, you don't have to do anything. It is perfectly okay to leave it alone. However, some blockages are particularly problematic so you need a method for releasing what has become stuck inside you.

Outer and Inner Dissolving

Although the Outer and Inner Dissolving processes are part of the same circle, the Inner Dissolving process is initially more difficult to do than the Outer Dissolving process.

The first phase of the Outer Dissolving process initially works with only the first two energy bodies, the physical and energetic. It is best used to mitigate or fully resolve problems in the physical body. The Inner Dissolving process works with the first seven energy bodies (see p. 76), a more complex task.

The Outer Dissolving process does not require you to have a sense of the motion of the mind or the Mindstream.[1] The process does, however, create an environment in which you may gain practical experience of the mind's normal motion first and, possibly, the significantly subtler Mindstream later. Whether you are deliberately looking for mind and Mindstream, they will be found. The Outer Dissolving process, along with the other preparatory practices, also usually creates "the wonderful accident" in which you can spontaneously encounter consciousness itself. For this reason, it makes sense to start practicing the Outer Dissolving process before moving on to deeper Inner Dissolving training unless you are an experienced meditator. A cornerstone of Taoist philosophy is grounding and starting your practice in your physical body.[2]

Letting Go Externally and Internally

The phrase used to describe the Outer Dissolving process has, for millennia, been "ice to water, water to gas." *Ice* refers to blocked, congealed energy; *water* refers to the accepting and relaxing of your internal blockage until it no longer causes you tension. *Gas* refers to the complete release of all the bound energy moving away from your physical body. The energy might revert to ice if the release is incomplete.

In contrast, the phrase used for the Inner Dissolving process of the Water method is "ice to water, water to space." *Space* refers to the vast internal space inside the body, space as infinite as the universe.

---

[1] The stream within which the totality of the mind, both conscious and unconscious, travels.

[2] This book, and Taoist meditation in general, concerns Inner Dissolving. The techniques described by the author are suitable for both novices and experienced meditators. These include various qigong practices incorporating Outer Dissolving, such as those in the author's book, *Opening the Energy Gates of Your Body*.

In the ice-to-water phase of Outer Dissolving, the solid, bound and condensed energetic shape (ice) is released until it relaxes and reaches the surface of your skin (water). In the Inner Dissolving process, your bound energy is also released at the point of the blockage until it becomes relaxed, soft and amorphous (water). Water, however, contains the inherent capacity to recondense to ice.

"Liquid" energy can now move in two different directions. In the Outer Dissolving process, you release blocked chi from your skin to outside your physical body and then to the edge of your chi or etheric body or even beyond (water to gas). The previously condensed energy is now neutral, unblocked, shapeless and lacking cohesion.

When you move into the water-to-space phase of the Inner Dissolving process, you release all blocked content of your *felt* sensations by imploding your energy *into* the inner space that the condensed, blocked, energetic shape occupied, thereby converting your blocked energy into consciousness without content. This is a beginning stage of emptiness. The Taoist position is that there is as much internal space inside you as there is space in the whole external universe.

The Taoist position is that there is as much internal space inside you as there is space in the whole external universe.

Using the Inner Dissolving method to go ever deeper inside during sitting meditation, for instance, is like letting your dissolved energy open a door into a door within a door, leading deeper and deeper into inner space, the point at which you began dissolving. You implode each layer of energy inward into the point, however far it extends internally, until you finally reach a place where your being naturally comes to a stop. This process may proceed very slowly and take a long time.

Depending on your individual nature, you might experience this endpoint as complete and utter yin or yang energy, a feeling or vision of light, or a sense of water, emptiness, calmness, peace or the mind expanding. Rest within that endpoint and try to develop the ability to return to that spot through all of the layers of your energy at will, especially in the midst of life's most scary and stressful situations. Eventually, if you dissolve deeply enough into any one spot, you will end up at your true consciousness, which, you will discover, has been relieved of the source of your blockage. Consciousness is permanent, and this is the exact point at which you have a glimpse—whether temporary or permanent—of consciousness itself.

 ## Personal Practice Session 8

Touch the very top of your head and find the exact middle— the place that was soft when you were a baby. This is the place where you should always begin your practice because all the yang energy forces in your body culminate here.

Start by putting your attention on the four conditions: strength, tension, something that doesn't feel quite right or some type of contraction. See them; feel them; taste them; listen for them. Become aware through whichever sense you can—everybody becomes aware in a different way. At first you may only be aware of your thinking, but then something more happens. Maybe it's a feeling deep inside your body. Later you may become aware of a feeling deep inside your heart and you begin to recognize ever more subtle layers. Just watch the process unfold and keep your attention and intention—your willingness—focused on staying present to what is happening. You don't have to do anything but keep your attention and intention on letting this blockage relax. You are actively waiting. You don't force the blockage to relax. You simply wait for the willingness for it to happen until it finally does.

Now choose a hand and let it be very relaxed. After a minute or two, squeeze it really hard [3] until your knuckle

---

[3] CAUTION ADVISED: If you have heart disease or very high blood pressure you are advised not to do this exercise as it may strain your body, a risk you don't need to take. ♥

turns white. That's ice. After a while, when the blood stops flowing, your hand will tingle and eventually go numb. This is one example of what a blockage might feel like in your body.

Next, put your intention on your hand. Let your mind focus on your hand and then, with your hand still in a fist, let it relax. Allow your hand to relax until all the feeling and blood comes back. This process can take a while. The more you hold on, the less you can let go and the longer it will take. The more you let go, the faster your hand will relax. Keep your hand in a fist. It's easier to relax your hand when you open it up, but the sheer act of making a fist is hard-wired into people to cause tension. When people get really angry they don't open their hands, they close them. If you were to try holding a fist for half an hour, you would see how exhausting it would become. It takes a lot of energy and stamina to maintain control and tension, yet people do it all the time.

Open your hand very slowly. See if you can let go of control and just let it open of its own accord. Don't try to control the movement of your hand; just let all the crinkles release on their own. As you let your fist release and the blood slowly comes back, your hand will open up. It may open up very slowly, but even so let it happen of its own natural accord. Let go of your need to control. If you can do this consciously, in time you can let go of the things you don't even know you were holding on to and you'll notice that you are more relaxed.

Author-guided Practice Session 5

Try the fist exercise: see p. 167.

Let Go, Chi Flows

We live in such a hurry-up-and-wait, exhausted, sleep-deprived society because people hold on to their tension. Most people don't know how to let go even when they want to. Whatever we hold on to that isn't real or necessary has a tendency to make us miserable. This is why letting go has such a powerful effect on human beings.

The Dissolving and letting go process is about dealing with both the things you know about and the things you don't. The human body has an energy field that works in a specific way. The Taoist tradition of China studied how people can make the central nervous system relax. Taoists created diagrams to explain the energetics of the body. They called this phenomenon *chi*, or your vital life-force energy (see p. 71).

Having chi means the difference between being physically alive instead of dead. In Sanskrit it was called *prana* and in Hebrew, *ruha*. Chi, prana and ruha are variously translated as breath, energy and spirit. The Taoists were particularly interested in understanding the nature of energy in the body and what allowed people to let go rather than remain stuck. They discovered that chi travels through the nerves. Chi also makes fluids such as blood move in the body, but when the nerves of the human body can't let go, chi becomes blocked. When our energy becomes unblocked, we can let go and relax.

So how do you let go of your nerves? How do you get the energy flowing so your body can work properly and your muscles and nerves can relax? How do you go into the depths of your mind and discover the energy that powers your emotions? The Dissolving method was developed to help you find these answers. When your energy flows freely, everything else goes with it. Everything else can let go. You can relax.

Personal Practice Session 9

Again, start at the top of your head and release what you can at any place where you find a blockage. If you find anything you can't release, move on and keep going down. Progressively scan down your body to the next place, the next blockage. Join everything together from the head down to that point and release once again: ice to water, water to gas. Don't worry about what you can't find—just work with what you can. Trust your awareness. Trust yourself because all human beings have intelligence within them. The deeper you go into your inner world, the more you release.

Begin slowly so that each layer of your nervous system, each layer of your mind, can release. If you do, it becomes easier to cross the barrier from focusing on the external world to focusing on what is inside you. You are developing a skill that, like any new skill, requires a learning curve. Eventually, you will train yourself how to let go. Letting go is a gift that was given to the human race. Life becomes a burden when you are stuck and strained.

When you finish practicing letting go with your eyes closed, especially if you have concentrated a little too much or your breathing wasn't smooth and continuous, the blood can get stuck in your head. To make sure your energy and blood don't get stuck in your head, rub your hands together until they become warm. Place them on the top of your head, right on the crown. Then slowly bring your hands down your face, down past your nose to your chin, down your throat and right down to your chest. Do this once or twice to help you bring the blood out of your head. You can also use this technique after you've been concentrating for prolonged periods, such as when you are on the computer. The purpose is to move chi out of your head and back into your body where it belongs.

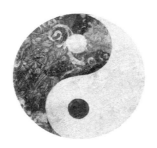

CHAPTER 6
Deepening Your Dissolving Practice

E veryone has a physical body. Energy runs it and emotions arise from it. The theory of Chinese and other forms of Eastern medicine is one of equivalence. For example, anger is associated with the liver, fear is associated with the kidneys and anxiety is associated with the heart. Each internal organ will produce certain types of emotions depending on whether they are working poorly or functioning optimally. We can call these emotions instinctual. If the internal organs are compromised, they can elicit negative emotions; if they are in top condition, they will produce balanced or smooth emotions. If someone is continually angry, the effect could work in the opposite direction, causing damage to the liver rather than a damaged liver causing the anger. Likewise, an overly anxious person can have a heart attack. It's a negative feedback loop.

The Value of Outer Dissolving

The Outer Dissolving process is good for making you physically healthy and balancing your internal organs. As your organs perform better, the corresponding instinctual emotions improve. If a person is diseased, specific organs are likely to be very weak and certain emotions are associated with those impaired organs. For example, sufferers of cirrhosis of the liver or hepatitis can be prone to anger.

Someone who has liver problems as a result of alcohol abuse is likely to have a short fuse—the raging drunk is a well-known cultural stereotype.

The Outer Dissolving process releases the chi inside your physical body, energy channels and aura (or etheric body). Moving from "ice to water" relaxes you, releasing blockages within the acupuncture points of your body, which are connected to the aura outside you. In effect the aura can be considered your external skin, enveloping your body. The inside of your body is what is underneath your skin. To deal with physical illness and generalized stress that can damage your body, the Outer Dissolving process is applied.

The Value of Inner Dissolving

The more experience you have with meditation, the easier it will be to comprehend the full value of the Dissolving process. Taoism, Buddhism and the Hindu yogic traditions more or less share this methodology of working with consciousness. This is the way in which Samadhi, or "absorption into the absolute," is accomplished in yoga. In a like manner, the water-to-space concept is used in Taoism.

To meditate using dissolving, the observer "I" first focuses his or her attention either on a physical object, whether outside or inside the body. The focus can be on emotional, mental, physical or psychic phenomena. It can come in the form of a feeling, ghost or image. From the interaction between the observer (subjective viewer/seer) and the observed (object/blockage), meanings or interpretations arise. The meaning often becomes more refined. Each interpretation can yield a more expanded realization of the interconnections between your object and everything that is tangential to it—no matter how subtle—until finally, in your mind, the meanings wash away. Even the object "dissolves" or, in yogic language, becomes absorbed until you go from water to space and everything becomes empty.

At this point your awareness is flowing steadily toward the object in an unbroken, nondistracted fashion so that the energy of the object unravels and breaks up. You subsequently become cognizant of what has occurred. As this disintegration happens, any attachments you have to the object also break up so that you resolve and embrace all the meanings of the object. The freed energy converts to spirit as you begin to move from water to space.

Then the meaning "drops" or "dissolves," and only you, the observer, remain. As you keep on dissolving, the sense of "I" (the observer), dissolves and you attain an inward stillness in which neither the form of the object, its meaning, nor a sense of yourself impinges on your complete awareness of consciousness itself. Prior to this moment, you have ignored your consciousness, which happens when you are internally blocked or cut off. Or you have been completely absorbed with some aspect of the content attached to your consciousness—the object's external form, meaning, interpretation or a sense of self. Each state of stripping this content increases the "mind's emptiness of content."

Ultimately, at the successful conclusion of the Samadhi/absorption or ice-to-space process, you achieve freedom from all the energetic and psychic attachments that bind and torture your body, mind and spirit. With that freedom, a release that allows your body, mind and consciousness to be totally at ease and comfortable is imbued with a spontaneously arising natural sense of inner stillness, quiet, peace and joy.

What Should I Let Go Of?

Many of my students ask me: "How do I know what to let go of, and how do I know what's holding me back inside?" The classic Chinese phrase is: "First learn to master yourself, next your family, then the world." Many people mistakenly think that their mentor, guru or some sort of God surrogate can give them the secret. But only you can ultimately discover what holds you back.

Meditation teachers who might actually know the answer may never say it flat out. They will only guide you to look inside until you find it for yourself because the only way human beings become free is when they discover their internal truth on their own.

Cutting the Root of an Agenda

One application of the Dissolving method uses agendas. Anything you need to do or stop doing can be an agenda. For example, you want to be more compassionate towards others, you want to communicate better with a family member or you want to find a career path that truly suits you.

The first question to uncover the truth is: What is holding me back? If you take this primary agenda, you will likely come up with at least two, three, four or 500 subsequent ones. When you've gone through those 500 agendas, all of a sudden it's going to become terribly obvious that there is yet another agenda emerging. If you were to swim from the surface of the ocean to its deepest recesses, it would take quite awhile. At every depth, the world would seem entirely different. When a human being follows the agendas until they cease, clarity emerges. There will be no doubt—just peace of mind. In essence, you are going to the energy behind, the energy behind, again and again, until you cut the root. And there, you will see there is nothing to do. No agenda.

Applying the Mind's Intent

In the Dissolving process, how does your mind contact, and then dissolve, the tension or blockage in your body? How can you deliberately contact, become aware of and feel the blockages in your body with your mind only? People with normal nerves will feel pain if you hit them forcefully in a sensitive body part. Sometime later they will feel the blockages inside their body as a throbbing pain. Likewise, a person can be erotically stimulated in a sensitive spot and feel pleasure. In strong emotional situations—such as falling in love, experiencing the death of someone close to you or being frustrated with situations beyond your control—you can consciously feel your emotions, positive or negative. With a little bit of concentrated "mind effort," you can increase, decrease or mitigate your physical pain, pleasure or emotions.

In externally induced situations, your whole mind concentrates and all your attention is drawn to the "object" at hand—be it pain, pleasure or emotion. The totality of your awareness, the "subjective observer," is directed at this object. The mind must be focused and not scattered or distracted. For instance, consider a baby that has fallen down some stairs and has real pain that would normally keep it crying for 10 to 15 minutes. The mind is fully focused on the pain. Every parent knows that if you can distract the baby with something more absorbing than the pain, the attention can be diverted to a new object, such as a favorite toy. Chances are that the baby will stop crying and focus on the new object. If, within a few minutes, you withdraw the toy, the baby will again feel the pain from the fall and will often resume crying again. Where did that pain go and from where did it return?

The answer is that the pain didn't go anywhere. The mind did. It takes a certain minimum percentage of your mind's capacity to be consciously aware of anything. When dissolving a blockage, your recognition or interpretation of what you are observing, along with your feelings, affects you, the observer. By going deeper and deeper inside the blockage toward its source, your mind moves further away from the original surface point of contact with the blockage and toward the root, where it can ultimately be fully resolved.

Beyond Past, Present and Future

Once upon a time, people lived by seasons. The insanity of modern life is time. In ancient times, deadlines were over weeks and months, not days. Then came the age of machines and, with it, pressure. Time is money. Time is life.

When you go deep into your inner world, amazingly all time is the same. In the depths of your mind, there is no

The insanity of modern life is time.

such thing as past, present or future. The natural state of the depth of the mind, the depth of the soul, is timeless because it's beyond past, present and future. In Sanskrit they call this *turia*. The Taoists call it *Fourth Time*: beyond past, present and future—the eternal now—or "real time."

Fourth Time is the state of mind you want during meditation because the mind cannot truly resolve what is at its depths by working within the normal idea of time. Yet obviously, even if you meditate, you also have to be able to function within "normal time," which includes past, present and future, in order to do things in the external world.

Your emotions, mental and psychic thoughts, karma and sense of satisfaction with life do not operate within time, even though everything else does. So your inner world—even when you meditate—needs to function within Fourth Time, beyond past, present and future. When ideas or energies appear inside you, there is no need to place them in time. Just let them be there. They will either get resolved or they won't.

 # Personal Practice Session 10

When you go back to the top of your head and start dissolving again, you want to look for, and dissolve within, Fourth Time. Look for the place where all time is the same—not past, not present, not future. Starting from the top of your head, move from blockage to blockage, going into each one, relaxing it and then completely letting go. Ice to water, water to space.

As you scan downwards, consider that everyone has courage inside. When you feel places that are stuck, you will need some courage to be willing to deal with that blockage.

Touch the very top of your head and find its exact middle. It will be on a line between your ears and your nose and the back and front of your head, right in the middle. Can you feel anything blocked inside you that your awareness can attach to? You are looking for one of the four conditions: strength, tension, something that doesn't feel quite right, especially if you don't know what it is, or any type of contraction.

Focus on that spot and just stay there for a while without the need to move on to other places in the body that may call out for attention. Instead, focus on whether you feel one of the four conditions in this spot or in the area surrounding it. Ice is not free, flowing or smooth. It's not like air. Something is not quite as it should be. Very often, this will be a vague sensation or feeling to you. You won't necessarily have a set of words to describe the sensation or feeling. And there is a sort of familiarity when that sensation or feeling arises. Put your attention on that area and let your mind be gentle. Be willing for it to soften. Maybe you will feel a buzz. It won't be soft and comfortable. Keep your attention on the blockage until it relaxes and becomes soft. Let go enough so that which is hard becomes soft, and relaxation will follow.

Beyond Ordinary Conscious Thought

If you just did the scan, going down through every part of your body, piece by piece, section by section, bit by bit, you would become physically relaxed. Physical relaxation is beneficial, but it will not take you to the depths of your mind, emotions and soul. In fact, it will not even take you into the depths of your central nervous system so that you can completely relax your nerves. Feeling better is not the same as completely releasing something. It's a great start, but much more is possible.

There is a barrier between ordinary conscious thought and the deeper levels of the mind. No matter how complex the thought, it still exists on the surface of your mind. When you go deeper, you may need to go through a subtle barrier in order to feel what your nervous system is really doing. When you reach this point, no matter how subtle an emotion is, you can feel its effects. If your inner world is out of balance, you will feel a sensation in the body. You can sense it. You can recognize it. You may see pictures or start talking in your head about it, but all of this is a distraction.

 ## Personal Practice Session 11

Again, start at the top of your head and as you scan downwards notice if any of the four conditions are present. Go to what is behind that energy. Follow the physical sensations and energy inside. Follow the energy through the layers.

You will become more aware of your nervous system, the nerves and the stress of your body and what is underneath it. As you go through the nerves, mind and spirit into the depths of your soul, follow the energy that is behind the place you have reached and just keep being willing to let go. As a blockage lets go, there will be something behind it, a sense of energy. Don't worry about any conversations in your head because they don't mean anything. It's what's behind the internal dialogue, what is below it, that keeps the blockage alive.

Where is the place from which your billions of thoughts arise? Follow it inside. Keep going. As you go deeper into the layer of the blockage, a sense of relaxation will show you yet another layer of tension. More ice. Let it melt into water and continue going deeper inside. Allow yourself to relax and let go. As you let go in that spot on the crown of your head, you will find that your whole body relaxes. Your whole body will open up to your awareness so that you become a being you know rather than a stranger. Rather than merely thinking about your body, you will actually feel it.

As you feel another layer of tension, again, just go into it. Be willing for the blockage to release and let it go, and you will move in deeper. Follow the energy that is behind it and do not get distracted by the thoughts, pictures or talking in your head, or by your interpretation of what you are feeling. Keep feeling. If you focus on interpreting too much, you won't go to the next, deeper layer. Eventually you will find a deep enough place inside you where that willingness for everything to release will happen. All of a sudden, you will feel as though you are completely letting go and what is inside you is expanding. You uncover the space inside you—the sense where you don't have "I" or "me," just space. In that space, there is life.

 ## Author-guided Practice Session 6

Look for Fourth Time and dissolve in this space: see p. 167.

Freedom Is Space

Usually, if you get to the point to where you release, you feel good for a while. If you have felt compressed, crushed or bound inside, you will feel an enormous sense of freedom when you get a release because you are no longer tied up in a straightjacket. For example, what you release may allow the blood in your arms to flow a little better so that you can move them around more easily and your range of motion is increased. You may release an old memory stored somewhere in the body that has the same result. You may not actually know what has caused the release, but you notice you feel better.

If you don't get a major release, that's fine. Just continue relaxing and sinking your intent into the blockage. Whenever you find any ice, turn it to water. Sometimes to get this release—which, when it happens very powerfully, is what in the East is called emptiness—everything loses all form. There is no more form. You have arrived at the essence of something. The essence is relaxed where nothing is anything in particular. Space is not an object. It is not something you can hold on to. It's just space. There is freedom in that space. It could take you weeks, months or even years to get there. And that's fine.

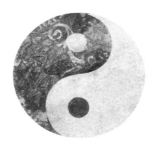

CHAPTER 7
The Descending Current of Chi: From Heaven to Earth

A fundamental principle of energetic training in the East, virtually unknown in the West, is that the energy moving from above to below is basically responsible for general well-being.

Ascending energy, which arises from the earth, is responsible for causing phenomena to occur and transform, and thereby raises human beings to a higher energy level than their original genetic capacity would dictate at birth.

Descending energy comes down from the cosmos through the human body to the earth. Its purpose is to release all energy the body cannot functionally use. Just as our body releases unusable toxins—including feces, urine, sweat, lymph and the out-breath—downward, we also release toxic or blocked energy down into the ground.

Similarly, the ascending current brings energy up the body in the same way an in-breath goes up our nostrils. If a wire (nerve) is not prepared to take a strong electrical current, damage—burnout, singeing, shorting out—can occur. The downward current clears the weakness in the wire, creating insulation, to accommodate the ascending current and save the nervous system from possible harm.

From the Chinese Taoist or Indian yogic viewpoint, it is not difficult to develop plenty of energy. The difficulty lies in creating a system strong enough to use this current safely and productively.[1]

When energy is flowing evenly, powerfully and naturally through you, you will experience a sense of comfort, ease and relaxed clarity. Blockages create sensations, which feel either positive or negative. Regardless, they are all essentially experiences of energy blockages. If the blockage feels bad, a person wants to "work through it" and a sense of achievement comes from emptying the garbage.

The sense of well-being and clarity that comes when energy flows smoothly does not have the incredible power surges and larger-than-life quality that many imagine. Rather, it is a very natural ease and connectedness, not only to yourself but also to your normal interactions in life and to your physical, mental and spiritual bodies.

Targeting Specific Blockages

As energy flows down, it is meant to be connected. If you are working on dissolving a blockage in your chest and then suddenly your attention goes to a blockage in your belly, you can be sure your energy is disconnected. As you release blockages, you want to maintain a sense of the downward flow. If the connection is not maintained, the effectiveness of your practice session will be greatly diminished.

Let's say you feel a blockage at the tip of your nose. If you make a ring around your head at the level of your nose, it would extend around to your cheek, your ear and to the top vertebra of your neck. Everything is at this one height. Imagine you are immersing yourself in a large pool of water. As you sink into the pool, every place the water touches makes a circle around you at the same height of your body. At any one of these levels, you could have a number of blockages. You might only have one at the tip of your nose; but, then again, you might have another at your ear, another at the back of

---

[1] To cultivate, store and move chi, the author recommends qigong or neigong training in conjunction with your sitting meditation practice.

your neck and yet another somewhere along the line of your jaw. There are a number of possibilities.

If you start the Inner Dissolving process—ice to water, water to space—you may find that the first blockage is at the tip of your nose. If you get a resolution, that's great. However, you may feel that you can release the blockage from ice to water but not to space. So you still have blocked energy in the tip of your nose, and your mind starts calling attention to one of the four conditions in your ear. At that point, using your attention and intention, you move all the energy you've brought into the nose to resolve the blockage there over to your ear. You do this to whatever degree your consciousness is capable, which will change from day to day and moment to moment. So, whatever did not release into space and is still water—or in the worst-case scenario, ice—gets combined with your ear. If there is one unit of energy blocked at your nose and two units at your ear, you now have three units of blocked chi at your ear. That is how much blocked energy would be at your ear. Then you repeat the process until, at some point lower down in the body, all the previously unresolved energy releases into space or emptiness.

Now let's say you had another blockage in the back of your neck. If you released into emptiness what was at your ear, you would just move to the back of your neck. However, if you couldn't release the ear blockage, then you would move its energy to the blockage at the back of the neck. Then start the whole process again—ice to water, water to space—and go down your body to notice the next place you have a blockage. It could be on the front of your face, back of your face, side of your face or in your neck. Even if the blockage had not finished releasing in the back of your head, you still would let that energy move to the next blockage lower in your body regardless of its location. Again the Dissolving process starts.

Your Intuition Is the Guide

Do your best to sit with a blockage. If at first it won't release actively, wait with relaxed intent.

If for any reason you cannot clear the blockage, you will have to leave it and come back to it another time. You don't want to apply any force, as this will result in diminishing returns. Straining to achieve a result is in direct contrast to the process of dissolving.

Do your best to sit with a blockage. If at first it won't release actively, wait with relaxed intent.

At any particular height-level in the body—it doesn't matter whether you move to the left or to the right, clockwise or counter-clockwise—keep following your intuition. A blockage will attract your attention like a magnet. As in your daily life, when something is stuck inside you, say a sore muscle, you are repeatedly drawn to that muscle even when you try to focus elsewhere.

As you practice more dissolving, your mind will move from the surface to the core of a blockage; it's like moving from the outermost ring of a dart board towards the bull's eye. You will likely find that you most easily penetrate the outermost ring of the blockage. As you develop your skill, you dissolve deeper inside yourself and your mind can enter into your body and energy field more deeply. You become capable of entering the center of a blockage. You start on the outer circle of the target and gradually, over time, you work on the next ring and then the next, until you eventually reach the core of your being.

Begin at the top of your head and move down your body, releasing what you can as you go downwards. When you find a point that you could work on dissolving for five minutes or the next 10,000 years but you know it's simply not going to fully release, then transfer that energy to the next blockage. The next blockage can be at the same height. But if everything else is free and open, go down to the next lower place in your body. Continue moving down until you reach your lower tantien, which is located in the middle of your body, about one-third of the way between your belly button and the top of your pubic bone (see p. 71).

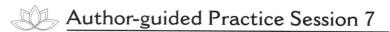 ## Author-guided Practice Session 7

Dissolve downwards: see p. 167.

Penetrating the Core of a Blockage

When you first start meditating, you will find that your ability to go inside your body, recognize a blockage and dissolve it is surface-level. Imagining a dart board going around and into your body in concentric circles, or a pool of water you have been immersed in up to the height of a blockage, start from the outer ring of the target. When you finally arrive at the point—the bull's eye—where you can release into inner space, just stay there for a while. It feels good because whenever a blocked energy force inside lets go, an expanded sense of wellness usually follows.

However, another possibility may occur that requires you to meditate for some time. When everything seems to settle down, all of a sudden a stirring inside emerges that signals something yet deeper inside the same blockage. Again, you will feel one of the four conditions that help you recognize this blockage. At the moment it starts to stir, you want to try to dissolve it.

Typically, if it takes you five minutes to as long as a half an hour to get a release, this next one could take a lot longer. When you start having a second release, you go to a much deeper place in your body where that blockage is attached. You are essentially going to a deeper root inside you that has not allowed you to fully let go. Easy blockages let go fairly easily, but core issues take a lot more effort to deal with.

Stay with it and don't use force. It's the same with everything in life—it's easy to let go of something that is not very important to you, but hard to let go of something that is. Use the power of your attention and your mind's intent to stay willing and open, and the release will come.

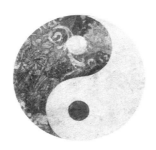

CHAPTER 8
How to Train the Monkey Mind

W hen starting meditation practice, many of my students tell me that their mind keeps wandering and they can't stay focused. This is a common problem in the twenty-first century. A relaxed mind can stay focused; a tense mind cannot. Go back to the fist-tightening exercise from Chapter 5. Try it again. This time, just see how long you can keep your fist tight. Can you last half an hour? You won't be able to do it. Tension saps your ability to focus and get anything done.

Calming the Monkey

Today, everyone multitasks. The MP3 player or television is on while you are at the computer, talking on your cell phone and having lunch all at once. The mind splinters into pieces. As this happens, your nerves become scattered, you become fragmented and rendered incapable of being present to your experience. Each time your mind jumps and swings from tree to tree, it's because you cannot be present to what is happening. The monkey mind is a symptom of the inability of the spirit to be comfortable. It's also a symptom of the body's energy being erratic, and it's habit-forming. The drive towards tension and the inability of the mind to stay still comes from not knowing how to relax and let go. The less peace you have inside, the more your monkey mind jumps around. So let go into some sort of inner peace.

For thousands of years, meditation practitioners have found that the process of calming the monkey mind is like breaking a wild stallion. When you first get on the horse, you have to stay with him because he bucks, sometimes really hard. You have to relax enough to have the wherewithal to stay with him. When you go into a blockage, you are going to the core of its energy. You are with it, you are with it, you are with it—and then you suddenly get thrown off. So you get back up and head back in again as if you were a surfer. You go out and catch the next wave.

When you meditate, every wave is different. First you play on the surface of the waves until you can start moving deeper and begin riding with the waves under the surface. You go down into the deep ocean to the place the surface waves originate. You again smooth things out a bit more. As you go deeper and deeper into the ocean, at every depth it's a whole different world. Meditation is not boring if you stay with it. When you stay with it, you let go and get used to moving into the space. You start feeling free. It's truly a gift of life to feel free.

Distraction after Clearing Blocks

After you go from ice to water, water to space, it's very important that you don't let yourself get distracted. Allow whatever is going on to continue of its own accord. The energy behind the energy is there inside you. Leave alone that which is external while you meditate. Let everything be as it is. This is the path to peace.

After having found some sort of blockage when going from ice to water, water to space, it is extremely common for people to become distracted and space out. All of a sudden, they wake up and they wonder what just happened. Even though people feel that they are spacing out or that their mind is wandering, they usually have actually gone to some interior space inside their mind. The experience is literally an unconscious daydream, and many people don't even know they had one, just as many don't consciously remember their sleeping dreams. You may have been dissolving something to do with a wonderful or horrible event in your life, and the input is so strong you cannot take it. Without you realizing it, you jump into a safer place within your mind. This place may be replete with beautiful green fields or loving situations.

Some people, however, cannot handle feeling too good. They cannot easily be happy, joyful or comfortable with themselves because deep down inside they feel that there is something fundamentally wrong with them. These people usually also avoid the situation and go into denial. They go to their version of a safe place in their mind where they can experience how dreadful they believe themselves to be. Whether you go to a place that is pleasant or awful, you lose your focus and don't consciously know you have done so.

When you snap out of it, you might feel completely spaced out and disoriented. Most likely you started telling yourself a story, and by the fourth or fifth chapter of this very long novel, you have completely forgotten the story line, or where you were going when you were dissolving. At this point, you want to start from the top of your head and dissolve downward once again if you cannot figure out where you left off.

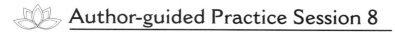 ## Author-guided Practice Session 8

Keep from getting distracted: see p. 167.

Dissolving a Psychic Itch

When you are dissolving, a particular place may start to call attention to itself. Let's say you are in the middle of your chest and all of a sudden a feeling around your eye or your nose starts becoming incredibly strong, demanding your attention. Some sort of a psychic itch crops up and you want to scratch it. The best possible thing you can do is *not* to give into the urge, even if it is driving you crazy. Continue dissolving downwards. Very often, when you reach a lower place in your body—maybe somewhere in your lower tantien—that other itch will suddenly resolve itself. You won't know why or how. This is the most likely scenario.

If, however, you decide to dissolve your psychic itch, you must re-dissolve everything you previously did below that point. So, if you have this itch in the middle of your forehead when you are at your belly button, you would have to dissolve everything in your body from your forehead down to below your belly button to receive the full value. You don't need to do this extra work. If you're already at your belly button and feel a psychic itch in your forehead, it isn't necessary to go back because all the energy in your body is connected like a hologram. It is not linear. It is not that A connects to B, which connects to C, which connects to D. Every point in your body is connected to every other point in your body.

Acupuncture provides good evidence of the body's complete interconnectedness. You have a pain in your knee, but the doctor may stick a needle in your ear to heal it. How is it that what is happening in your ear could have something to do with your knee? Resolutions do not always happen in the same place as they are started. If a giant river is poisoned at its source, you may not notice the poison until much farther downstream or where the river empties into the ocean. The source of the problem may be invisible. So you have to track backwards.

> *Every point in your body is connected to every other point in your body.*

The nature of the body as a hologram means that every single point where you feel a blockage is connected to every other place inside your body, your emotions and your thoughts. It is connected, directly or indirectly, to every one of these points. So it's very hard to tell while you are dissolving if something that you are feeling physically may actually be released by reaching a place deep in your mind until after it has occurred. Some physical issues are purely physical while others have subtle but clear emotional and mental components. Thus, the series of interlinked blockages you are dissolving may be maintained and unbroken, ultimately preventing the blockages in the middle from resolving. On the other hand, mental anguish may be relieved via a physical release in your body. The ancients found that logic alone could not bring resolution.

Sometimes a blockage can be released in one session—in one or two hours, or even in five minutes. Other times a deep blockage inside you can take months or even years to trace through all the secondary paths, all the little winding roads that block your energy, until the epicenter reveals itself. When you release the main point, you may never actually know what caused the blockage, but, in the process of releasing it, the system relaxes and all the consequences downstream vanish with it.

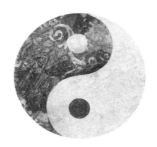

CHAPTER 9
Dissolving Emotions and Shock

Feeling Emotions below the Surface

If you practice trying to be aware of your emotions, you will learn how to feel ones that initially seem very weak. You will start to recognize when an emotion is not expressed strongly in response to a circumstance, but is like a seed that sprouts with the right amount of sunlight and water. So notice the energy of your emotions. On days when something makes you really angry, afraid, sad, greedy or anxious—anything for which you can point to an external cause—your emotions are easy to recognize. Some days no obvious emotion can be found, just a feeling of what an emotion is like when it's very, very subtle. In the following practice session, see if you can relax any of the four conditions that you find while putting your attention on your emotions. What does an emotion feel like?

 Personal Practice Session 12

Start at the crown of your head and for just a few moments start thinking about your emotions. Maybe you are angry, maybe you are sad. See if you can recognize what any emotional strength feels like. If you are feeling angry, stubborn or anxious it makes you feel strong in your

emotion. What does a sense of emotional tension feel like? Something inside you is fighting with something else. What does it feel like when something doesn't feel quite right emotionally, especially if you don't know what it is—or even if you do? What does an emotional contraction feel like when you are closing into yourself? Notice how these feelings are icy. Feel how you are blocked. Then put your intention and willingness into relaxing: ice to water, water to space.

Each time you find more tension or something not quite right, go deeper as the onion layers peel away. Feel what is a little deeper inside you and get a sense of what tension feels like. You may feel strength or a blockage. The energy is not smooth and maybe you feel a buzz from the continual firing of your nerves. It could also be a feeling of deadness. Maybe you just keep finding yourself spacing out. Once you have identified a source, a place that calls attention to itself, start going deeper into that point through the layers. What is the energy behind, behind and behind? Each time, relax deeper into that place. At times, you may get flashes of insight: "Oh, this happened. Oh, this is what that means. Oh, that is what this means." Just continue looking for the energy behind the sensation or a feeling you can recognize.

Distractions are tactics of the mind that prevent you from reaching your core. Just keep going and with any luck you will finally let go. A little letting go is into relaxation; a big letting go is into space. There is nothing but space inside you, an infinite amount of space. In that space there is freedom, in the sense that nothing binds you; all is as it should be. Something takes you back to that place inside you that everyone has, yet, unfortunately, most people rarely find. Only on occasion will you come back to the core of your being. Let go there; allow your experiences to integrate. Let everything inside your body and mind become familiar with this place, where there is space that you can have in your life any time, wherever you are.

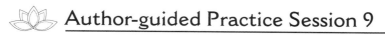 ## Author-guided Practice Session 9

Dissolve your emotions and shock: see p. 167.

Letting Go Begins with Your Intention

This is the process of Inner Dissolving: ice to water, water to inner space. The more you relax, the more you let go, the more clarity and balance will follow. All you need to take on the journey is your attention and your willingness to allow your awareness to settle inside you. Your intention to let go—not force, not your demand—will take you there.

As you get into the habit of letting go, it becomes easier to do. After you practice for a while—even in the midst of the most explosive situation in your life, if just for a few seconds—see if you can recognize any of the four conditions that might be present. You can let go immediately and enter the blockage with all your awareness. Your spirit becomes aware of where you are stuck and, like ice turning to water, you are willing to let go. You wait and, as long as you are willing, the blockage will eventually begin to release. You simply have to be willing and have the courage to encounter whatever you find.

All kinds of images will come up, images of real events and people, from computers, television, photographs, books and from your imagination. Let all those pictures that make your system tense break up and release. Let go of the vibration behind any words that come up, good or bad, or sounds that caught your attention. Let go of the sights and sounds of stored memories and emotions as they come up. Sometimes a vivid smell will even arise when you start relaxing. Maybe the memory was so deeply buried that you weren't conscious of it affecting you. Let it go. It doesn't matter how you experience the energy or what channel it is arising from. Just let it go.

The Courage to Practice

Dissolving on a regular basis releases all blockages, old and new. It is your cleansing process to release the tension that builds up in your body. When you have a 10-minute coffee break at work, instead of going for the caffeine, take five minutes to dissolve. Whatever the freak-out of the day is, it's best to release it from your system so you don't have to carry it for the rest of the day. Maybe something that happened at work triggers all the emotions that have been troubling your relationship for the past five years. If you take a few minutes during lunch to practice, you might be able to bring yourself back to your baseline. You don't need to be filled with continual giant floods of negativity. You can release any buildup and bring yourself into a more relaxed state.

After a rough day, instead of just sitting on the couch and watching television for two or three hours to calm your nerves, just take 20 minutes to dissolve so the rest of the night is yours. If you dissolve, you won't carry another layer of tension in your body and another layer of stress in your mind and emotions to the next day. Whatever you practice, you become—practice being tense and you will be tense; practice being stressed and you will always be stressed; practice letting go and in time you will be able to let go. As you let go of what stops you, you will discover that the space inside you is intrinsically balanced. It's balanced of its own accord. Compassion can completely fill that space, if only you have the courage to let it.

Dissolving Shock

One day, you may experience serious shock. If so, you need to know how to release it so that it doesn't attach to anything else inside you and create bigger problems. For example, if you suddenly have a large loss in the stock market, you want to dissolve the shock of learning most of your retirement has been squandered away. Otherwise, you may react from a position of fear and go on a mad selling rampage without sound reason, only to find that those stocks recover within a matter of days or weeks. Dealing with the shock becomes more complicated because it might become attached to regret for having made a rash decision by selling off. So it is best to dissolve shock as close to when it happens as possible, although you can make resolving previous shocks an agenda, which Chapter 11 will explain in detail.

Think back to when you had a serious shock in your life. See if you can remember the details. There are natural disasters, losses of loved ones, financial meltdowns, sudden injuries—tragedies happen all the time. Remember how, at that time, you were dazed and not present to the shock that befell you.

Start at the top of your head and, rather than being spaced out and incoherent, breathe into each area of your body that you get to as you dissolve downwards. Breathe until your awareness clears enough that you can be conscious of what is going on. Simply breathe into that part of your body so your awareness expands and you can stay present.

Take your time and when you're ready, begin dissolving. Dissolve down from the top of your head and, just as you did before, go through your body bit by bit. When attempting to deal with shock, you will have an even greater tendency to become distracted by thoughts, very strong feelings or even pain. No matter how bad these sensations are, you can start the Dissolving process.

You can release the shock at the moment you notice the blockage starting to take hold in your system. Simply breathe and dissolve. Let go: ice to water, water to space. Once dissolving and resolving the immediate shock begins, it often links and opens up other parts of unresolved shocks in your system. When this happens, you can include a new agenda: "I want to release, to get rid of the shocks I had when I was younger." If you can go back and release all the feelings associated with trauma, you become free from its burdens.

Shock makes it very difficult to be present. If you release the trauma stored within, you can be present once again. And being present to life—just as it is—is one of the greatest gifts.

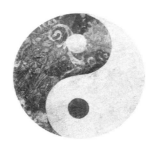

CHAPTER 10
Dissolving Fog and Depression

People get in a fog by not being present to the experiences of their lives. We can go through periods in life when we essentially fritter away our existence. We're only half there because of a mental or emotional state, because some accident has happened or for any of 10,000 other reasons.

People can go for years never getting anything done or having any idea what they want to do. They are lost, so they drift from one thing to the next without really having anything to care about. When the fog gets strong enough, it begins blocking out the ability to be present to almost anything. In any activity they do they are only half there.

Likewise, all meditators at some point or another experience fog in their practice. It's extremely common. Fog can be characterized by the feeling that nothing is happening. When you experience fog in meditation, you're not just having a boring time; it's a real experience. The only way to get rid of it is to dissolve it or actively cleanse your system of it.

A fog usually occurs not at the beginning of a meditation session, but somewhere in the middle. You may have been dissolving when all of a sudden you find yourself drifting. You might try to think about something, but you can't quite do it. Thoughts come into your head and they pass by without ever quite making any sense.

Taoism and Buddhism classify many different kinds of fog, but whatever the cause, the solution is the same: ice to water, water to space. Keep on dissolving the feeling behind the fog, feeling behind it layer by layer, until it goes away.

Deceptive Internal Dialogue

After a release, the mind has a tendency to wander. Every once in a while some sort of internal dialogue starts. You might start reciting a poem internally, or the words to a song, something from a laundry list, a conversation you had or something you have read in a book. Whatever it is, words will suddenly start coming up. You don't want to focus on interpreting what these words mean because they usually don't mean anything relevant to your agenda.

Instead, become aware of the energy behind the words, the energy that is generating them. Sometimes people see pictures or hear sounds inside their head. They are not going crazy and these are not hallucinations. The mind holds an incredible number of internal images, sounds, words, feelings, smells and sensations of touch. You experience them when you dream. You don't see with your eyes, you see with your brain. You don't hear with your ears, you hear with your brain. You don't feel with your skin, you feel with your brain.

The fact is that people confuse the sense organs that perceive with what is actually being perceived. Perception is in the mind. So words, sounds and pictures emerge, and the tendency is to get distracted

You don't see with your eyes, you see with your brain. You don't hear with your ears, you hear with your brain. You don't feel with your skin, you feel with your brain.

by them. When you meditate, notice the energy that comes up inside your mind. Yes, the monkey mind will try to distract you, but what is the feeling behind that energy?

As you go in further and deeper, sometimes words can suddenly take on a life of their own. Or, out of nowhere, you start wondering why you are experiencing a given memory that will distract you if you try to interpret it. If you can avoid this tendency and keep dissolving the energy behind the conversation, the pictures or sounds that arise, you may actually go much further towards the root of the symptom and release it. Even before you have a big release, you might experience an emptiness accompanied by insights into what the blockage is really about. Then again, you may not. Either way, no insight will arise from just thinking through and analyzing what is happening. Ninety-five percent of all the experiences you will have in meditation will mean nothing, but if you keep on going behind, behind, behind when you release, the blockage will be gone.

People tend to want to analyze their situation so they can come to a definitive conclusion about it. Yet to effectively deal with a blockage, you don't need to find out where it came from. You just need to know how to get rid of it. The ancients had a saying originating from a culture that allowed torture for thousands of years: "If you are on a torture table, would you rather know why you are being tortured or would you simply like to get off the table?" Forget *why* you're there and just get off the table.

Face or Happiness—It's Your Choice

The antidote to fog is being present and being able to allow what is to be. When we cannot allow what is to be, we are left miserable. My teacher Liu once said something that had a very profound impact on me: You can save face or you can be happy. That is, you can hold on to the feeling that your position is very right and justified—no matter how much pain or anxiety it may cause you—or you can let go of the burden of needing to be right, thereby giving you the freedom to be happy. The ability to let go of what you hold on to is very important, especially in the West where honor, pride, a sense of self-worth, looking good and identities—"I am this" or "I am that"—figure so prominently in our culture.

Fog, besides having the quality of drift, also has a quality of anger, frustration or greed. Most of the time it isn't quite clear which emotion lies beneath the fog. Maybe you experience a kind of general malaise and a feeling of being drained that goes on and on. In many countries where people have been in continuous warfare for a long time, they finally get to a point where they just give up. They don't want to die, but they don't want to live either. They are stuck in limbo.

What part of us, no matter how unconscious, needs to create fog? Fog makes us disengage from life, even though we don't want to. Fog protects a person against feeling anything that is too difficult or strong to handle, understandably so. Sometimes this is called burnout. Don't let yourself spend decades drifting in fog because you give up. Ice to water, water to space.

Depression Is a Black Hole

What is the difference between fog and depression? The quality they have in common is a disconnection from life. You are not willing to be alive, not fully alive, because for whatever reason reality has become too tough to face. The difference is that depression has a tendency to make people fall deeper and deeper into a dark hole where everything seems totally black.

When people become truly depressed, they go through every reason why life is essentially horrible and useless. Eventually they collapse internally. Using dissolving to deal with serious depression takes a great deal of work and may be very difficult unless the person has the courage to face their internal demons.[1] The depth of what can produce depression may be linked to the deepest corners of the soul.

 ## Author-guided Practice Session 10

Let go of fog and depression: see p. 167.

Let go of fog and depression: see p. 167.

---

[1] CAUTION ADVISED: People suffering from depression are advised to consult their licesnsed healthcare provider before embarking on the practices in this book. These practices are not recommended for those with severe depression.

Oh, You Think Life Is Fair?!

All kinds of blockages can be resolved by dissolving. The Taoists say that because the ghosts in your mind are not real, they don't have a right to inhabit the land of the living. Yet we allow them in all of the time. My teacher Liu responded to my complaints about my parents with, "Oh, you think life is fair?!"

A few days later, he told me I should meet someone he knew to be a very good meditator. This middle-aged man was taken in the Cultural Revolution and put into a torture camp.

> *Having a terrible event take place is bad enough. The really horrible thing is reliving any bad incident over and over.*

The warden was curious about how long he could keep a man alive if he tortured him twice a day. He tried this experiment on a few hundred people, including the man I spoke with. Nobody lasted past three months except this one guy.

When I met him, he was obviously very alive and happy. He had a depth in him that I've rarely seen in other human beings. When I had a discussion with him about compassion and human suffering, it went into every cell of my body. He told me that when the warden tortured him, he would dissolve as best as he could during the session. At a certain point he just couldn't continue, but the moment the warden let him go, he would start dissolving again, trying to release everything that was done to him. The man said he must have gone through at least 200 or 300 instances when he just wanted to give up and let the warden kill him, but he didn't. The issue is not that bad things happen. The issue is whether you choose to live with them forever or struggle for a period and eventually get rid of them. That's it.

The ghosts are only in your mind. They might be in your nervous system, they might be in your emotions, they might be in your psychic field—but they don't really exist. Nevertheless, it's one thing to know this as an intellectual comment; it's another thing to practice and clear the ghosts. Having a terrible event take place is bad enough.

The really horrible thing is reliving any bad incident over and over. It's not so much about what has happened to you, it's about whether you hold on or let go of it. Ice to water, water to space. When you can let go of what is bothering you, joy and happiness will naturally resurface.

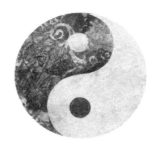

CHAPTER 11
Ten Thousand Agendas and the Greatest Poverty in Existence

In nearly three decades of teaching, the question of how to fomulate an agenda is probably the one most frequently asked. People can have many agendas. An agenda is anything you want to address because you know enough is enough and you want to be rid of it. The content of an agenda can be whatever you wish it to be. One application of the Dissolving method is to let go of whatever needs to drop away. You make whatever comes up in your life—no matter what it might be or how it is manifesting—into an agenda so you can dissolve it. This technique involves the way you move your energy. It starts by activating your intent.

Formulating an Agenda

If you want your mind to be magnetized toward a certain agenda, you need to contemplate it before you begin dissolving. If you do so during the day or an hour before you practice, it's usually enough. Or, you could focus for the next few minutes on the emotion associated with your agenda as you scan downward. You could also think about a specific situation that you're holding on to. Maybe you think about how someone lied to you, how you lost in a situation when you expected to win. Pick something and focus on it.

Now, you can go about this process in two ways. You can just keep on thinking about an emotion in general, or you can think about a particular issue that you have in relationship to that emotion—either way, you're formulating an agenda. It doesn't much matter because if your mind is focusing on a particular emotion, your energy will start moving toward where it is inside you. When you truly become free inside, you will no longer experience this pull.

Experiencing the full range of emotions is natural and healthy, but as your ability to dissolve agendas increases, you won't experience the spikes where you erupt in anger, burst into tears or jump for joy with little or no stimulus. You will just flow from one emotion to the next and your emotional response will be more proportional to the positive or negative experiences themselves.

When you start thinking about a particular emotion, rub or press against the corresponding organ to help make you aware of the ways in which emotions can also be a bodily experience. Fear is linked to the kidneys; anger is linked to the liver; grief is linked to the lungs; anxiety is linked to the heart.

Sit down and think about your agenda for 15 minutes before you start meditating. Think about why you hold on to this issue. After 10 minutes, let your mind completely relax. Let everything go out of your mind and just sit there and wait. At some point, you will get a very light sense of the emotions associated with your agenda, or at least some sense of stirring inside.

Start from the top of your head and dissolve down to the bottom of your belly. As you continue dissolving down from the top of your head, you are always feeling for the energy behind whatever comes into your awareness. Thoughts will come into your awareness and you may start talking to yourself. It's very important that you don't try to edit the thoughts. Stay with the energy behind them. Suddenly you can find yourself going into an entirely different space of your inner world than where you have ever been before. Let whatever thoughts, whatever conversations you are having in your head—the monkey mind jumping from tree to tree—come up, but keep aware of the energy behind these conversations. Keep dissolving and staying focused on the energy behind what you are feeling.

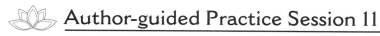 ## Author-guided Practice Session 11

Let go of your agendas and expectations: see p. 167.

The Beast of Greed

Greed, hatred, anger and fear are the four primary emotions connected to expectations. Greed is the constant expectation of more, more, more! The beast of greed inside human beings can never be satisfied. There is no limit to greed. The modern mantras are: "I consume, therefore I am; I want, therefore I am; I get, therefore I am." People are obsessed with acquiring more than they will ever use. Obtaining material goods is not a problem in itself; the issue is one of balance and what it does to the heart and soul. There is no rest from greed. It prevents people from being grateful even for a few moments when things are going their way. It doesn't matter what they get; it's never enough.

At the bottom of greed is a hole that cannot be filled. You may think that by getting what you want, you will fill that hole, but it doesn't work that way. Consider what greed does to you. It keeps you continuously spinning in a black hole because wanting something is not the same as having it. Greed eventually turns to anxiety, which will be discussed in detail in the next chapter. First you become anxious about whether you are going to get whatever it is that you are after. Then you become anxious about whether you are going to get enough of it. Next you become anxious about how you could lose it. These are the faces of greed.

Loneliness

Of course, greed can also be accompanied by hatred, jealousy or envy towards people who have what you want. How many valuable friendships have been lost to greed? Human relationships make life a real joy. Ask any wise person, especially as he or she gets older, what the true wealth in their life is, and they always say one thing: relationships. Loneliness and the lack of decent human relationships is the greatest poverty in existence.

If you feel that the need to acquire things is controlling your life to some degree, you might want to ask yourself: "What is greed to me? Do I want to be greedy? Where does this greed come from?" Really look into it. Any place you feel one of the four conditions, something stuck inside you, keep on following the energy behind, behind, behind, and slowly the greed will begin to calm down. Ice to water, water to space.

The Antidote to Greed

Taoists say it doesn't actually matter how much money, material goods or power a person has. There is a simple antidote to greed in terms of how it affects the soul. They say it is fine to have anything you want as long as you use it. It doesn't matter what you accumulate as long as you use it. Now for most things, you use them for a while and then you stop. When you find yourself no longer using something, get rid of it.

This antidote will help you to find real value in your life so you are not misguided in buying things you don't need, hoarding money you'll never use and running around like a hamster on his wheel. Can you recognize what in your life brings true value? Continually acquiring material things is not sustainable and feeds the need to replace them with newer, better items. Whereas anything that adds intrinsic value to your life will stay with you through the years. Once you can recognize and appreciate that which has value, you will cease chasing after the things you previously sought in the first place.

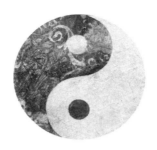

CHAPTER 12
Anxiety: The Disease of the Modern Age

We live in an age of anxiety, where the fast pace of modern life causes people to become overwhelmed. While intelligence obviously has its advantages, it can make you more inclined to think about how everything in your life can go wrong. Intelligence can be a curse at one level because it lends itself to more creativity in mentally conjuring up everything that could go horribly wrong. Of the billions of events that someone could imagine going wrong within the next hour, maybe one will happen somewhere in the world. Nothing—absolutely nothing—will protect us from the paranoia of our own minds unless we release the place deep inside us from which paranoia is born: pain. Pain likes pain. Misery enjoys miserable company.

When you feel overwhelmed and look at things in terms of the two, five, 10, 20 or 50 tasks you have to do as all having equal importance and priority in your mind, then each one starts driving you a little crazy. You could spend time prioritizing and putting some things on the back burner, but instead your mind cycles through the list repeatedly, adding more responsibilities along the way. It's a negative feedback loop. Your nervous system becomes involved trying to affect events it can do absolutely nothing about as you become obsessed by all the things you need to do. Staying on this rollercoaster causes pain. So look inside yourself and find the place deep in your mind that makes you predisposed to becoming overwhelmed, anxious and frustrated because you are trying to keep together more than is humanly possible. Ice to water, water to space.

The Energy of Overwhelmingness

For each block you find—whether it's strength, tension, something that doesn't feel quite right, especially if you don't know what it is, or any kind of contraction—how do you start going into it and letting it lead you to the place where the paranoia, fear and overwhelmingness reside? Letting that place take over can lead to paralysis and everything in your system shutting down. Or it can make you run around like a chicken with its head cut off, going everywhere but getting very little done. You waste an incredible amount of mental and emotional energy.

Life needs rhythms of rest and activity, but if you let your doomsday thoughts run in a continuous loop, there can be no rest. Your sleep is interrupted and you can't even sit and regenerate. Begin by simply looking inside yourself for the energy of being overwhelmed, the place that is always looking for things to go wrong. Follow the energy behind and further behind, releasing each layer before moving on to the next. There is a big difference between surviving and living. To be fully alive you have to go past being overwhelmed. If you can deal with something, deal with it. If you can't deal with it, don't beat yourself up because you are not a god who can do everything. Look for the place inside your soul where you simply let energy go so it doesn't build up and get stuck. Release it. Ice to water, water to space.

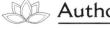 ## Author-guided Practice Session 12

Dissolve your anxieties: see p. 167.

The Mentality of an Overachiever

Achievement is good, but the mentality of an overachiever is one of never feeling that anything is enough. It won't matter what you achieve and what you keep on achieving because you are always going to find a way to punish yourself by going for more. How do you beat yourself up? What is inside your mind that tells you you'll be a failure if you don't achieve the something or another? What are the things inside you that you are driven to achieve? Overachievers very often only get one part of the equation. Since they are only looking for achievement, they don't consider the peace, joy and happiness that could be found. They lack balance. On the other hand, some people are real underachievers, and there can be a tremendous series of consequences to pay for not having goals.

Find the Joy that's Already Here

Where is the balance between getting things done and having a life worth living? If your insides tear you apart, it doesn't matter if you are the wealthiest and most powerful person in the world, or if you are the poorest and most wretched person in the world. You cannot escape what is inside you. You walk with yourself 24 hours a day, regardless of your external wealth, poverty, power or powerlessness. If you release the pressure and feeling of being overwhelmed, you stop beating yourself up. Immense joy will naturally arise inside you. You don't have to create it; it's already there.

What frustrates you? Why are you beating yourself up? How do you beat yourself up? Everyone has their own variation. Do you always have to win? Do you always have to lose? There are as many stories as there are people in the world. Rub your heart and notice if you feel any sensation, as anxiety affects the heart. Dissolve. Let go of how you beat yourself up. You are not helping anyone—especially not yourself. If you have done something you know is wrong, dissolve the blockages inside that stop you from recognizing it in its totality. Dissolve what stops you from recognizing how it affected everybody else downstream. Dissolve how it is affecting you until you arrive at genuine remorse because you recognize what you have done. Finally, dissolve and remove that remorse. If you truly have remorse and you go through to the end, fully comprehending what you have done, you create enough space to free yourself from ever doing it again.

When the pain that drives you to deny or to lash out disappears, you lose the need to engage in that behavior again. When people never experience remorse, even if they have an innate criminal mentality, they will find ways to punish themselves with self-inflicted pain. Will it be by overachieving? Will it be through the emotions of frustration or self-hatred? Some people believe in the convoluted argument, "Why let someone else punish me when I can use guilt to punish myself more than anyone else could?" Many people use a slow mental form of torture on themselves. Creativity can be magical, but it can just as easily cause unnecessary suffering. What do you need to reach the end, to release your pain, achieve clarity and recognize what you have done so that you can let go and change? Stop the cycle of self-inflicted pain. Ice to water, water to space.

> *If you truly have remorse and you go through to the end, fully comprehending what you have done, you create enough space to free yourself from ever doing it again.*

Perfection In Imperfection

Some ancient traditions, including Taoism, say that when you penetrate to the core you will recognize that everything is perfect. If it weren't perfect, it wouldn't exist. If you reach the point of spirituality and you become fully awake, you will see everything as essentially positive even if sometimes absurd. You will see how everything is in some way necessary and you simply will understand that life is perfect just the way it is.

Many people are preoccupied with trying to be perfect. We think our role models are all supposed to be perfect. But if you looked into the deeper layers of all the greatest human beings throughout history,

I guarantee you that none were perfect. According to any conventional perspective, maybe a piece of perfect inorganic matter can exist completely and utterly balanced, but absolute perfection cannot be achieved by a human being.

In the same way, many believe that human beings are supposed to be able to love everybody else and have compassion for all. Although that is a truly marvelous goal, have you met many people who can show compassion for everyone and everything in life? This ideal is certainly worth aspiring to. Nevertheless, attempting to be perfect in this way carries a burden. If you aspire to be perfect, you will think of yourself as unworthy until you meet your lofty goal. "I'm not perfect, I'm not worthy," may be the voice you hear in your head. Once you believe that you are unworthy, you give yourself the ultimate justification for messing up every part of your life.

Perfection drives people crazy and yet it has its good sides. The idea of being perfect, of creating the best possible outcome, is a reasonable goal. Yet for many of those striving for perfection, giving 100 percent is never enough—forget about 70 percent—even 150 percent won't be enough. Consider where perfection resides inside you. Where is the balance between doing your worst and putting forth your full effort without the strain?

The finest diamonds in the world all have flaws. Yet their beauty goes way beyond the flaws. We can grow perfect, flawless diamonds in laboratories, but somehow the beauty is lost. Something about our imperfections brings out our humanity.

At the purely mental level, which is actually the only place where perfection exists, wanting to be perfect but not becoming perfect becomes the pain of existing. Every human being who becomes completely awake and clear eliminates his or her pain of existence. The lack of freedom inside of human beings always creates a kind of pain because something is fundamentally missing. Nearly all the meditation traditions of the world—including the practices of Christianity, Judaism, Taoism, Islam and Buddhism—have observed that unless we have direct contact with the core of our being, we always have a sense of existential pain from the feeling that something is missing. When you become completely coherent and internally whole, that feeling will just go away of its own accord.

Finding Space with Clarity

Some people may be numb to their life force, but every spirit wants to be free. No amount of wealth, prestige, power, status or anything in the outer world can fill that hole. It can only be filled when the inside of a human being wakes up.

So make clarity an agenda. What prevents you from being clear? What prevents you from being awake? First

> *Some people may be numb to their life force, but every spirit wants to be free.*

take on the simple stuff—anger, fear, frustration—but eventually, the agenda has to be everything that prevents you from finding clarity and becoming awake. At that moment when you find it, you are free. Since the time many of us were children, we have wanted to understand why we are here on earth and what it's all about. Ultimately, finding the space of clarity inside you is the only answer.

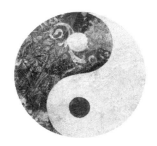

CHAPTER 13
Anger and Frustration as Agendas

There are millions of justifications for anger. Yet most people are not actually angry just because of the reasons or excuses they give. At one level we get angry for a very basic reason: We have a body. If you have glands, you have the potential for anger. If you have a liver, you have the potential for anger. The emotion won't go away unless you learn what to do with it. It is usually accompanied by heat and goes to the eyes. Have you ever noticed that when people are really angry, it's as if you can see their eyes from a half a mile away? They beam lasers at you. When the eyes alone cannot contain the anger your brain gets involved. When your brain cannot contain the energy, the emotion goes into your muscles. At this point, you may have what is colloquially referred to as a freak-out. You go mad. Your blood turns hot, you later regret the behavior that follows and you have to spend time apologizing for it.

Don't Wait for an Explosion

When you dissolve—ice to water, water to space—one of the first things you will notice is that some blockages will have a sense of anger attached to them. There may not be any fact, justification or story, just a sense of anger. It may be very quiet, like a radio dialed down to its lowest volume, or it can be as loud as an orchestra inside you. Anger is the most common distraction hindering you from being able to stick with the process of dissolving and letting go. When anger starts building, we start telling ourselves stories. We have to justify why we need to be angry. Within families, anger can easily spread like wildfire. One person gets angry and it jumps to the second person, third person and fourth person, and before you know it everyone is angry with somebody else. So if a story comes up, just for a moment, try to find the energy that is creating the story behind your anger. Keep on dissolving that energy: ice to water, water to space.

The stories you tell yourself can change. This is because every major blockage inside you is connected to the millions of other experiences that have something in common with that blockage. Maybe not in terms of the facts—the facts themselves are quite irrelevant—but rather in terms of the feeling, reaction or charge, whether negative or positive. Anger has a way of taking you over and making what is inside you vibrate or shut down. When you become angry, the facts become irrelevant—all you want is to continually justify one fact: that you are angry or, in an era when blame is common currency, that you are right. You end up saying things you don't mean and even things you do mean, but wouldn't normally say because they would hurt someone's feelings unnecessarily.

So as you track back to these stories that come up inside you, recognize when you find one of the four conditions and dissolve, ice to water, water to space. Often we don't recognize anger until it finally bubbles up to the surface after having linked to some blockage within us that needs to be addressed. Don't wait for the explosion—or implosion as the case may be—and then add guilt and other negative emotions that exacerbate the problem.

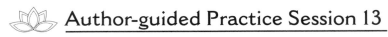 # Author-guided Practice Session 13

Dissolve anger and frustrations: *see p. 167.*

When Everyone Is the Enemy

Anger has three very clear phases: irritation, seething and the overt explosion or quiet implosion. By practicing meditation, you can recognize these qualities throughout your day and do something to head off anger. It is built into our physiology, so to completely obliterate anger you would have to remove your liver and a couple of glands. In effect, you would have to cease being human and become a robot without any feelings. And, from the Taoist perspective, you wouldn't want to because anger also has the positive quality of helping you take action. What do most people do if they are stuck and need to do something incredibly difficult that requires the force of will? They get angry. All of a sudden, in the righteous indignation of the full flowering of their ego, they somehow find the energy and the strength to take action.

In the days of cavemen, when a saber-tooth tiger wanted to eat you for lunch, you needed the power to get away or fight back. You couldn't become paralyzed or you would die. But there was a price to pay. Anger causes the glands in your internal organs to release poisons, which may leave you feeling terrible for days. You may get a headache, your blood may feel like it is boiling or you may feel sick. If King Kong were attacking your village, a giant tiger were chasing you down the street or a raving maniac were flashing a weapon at you, then it might be well worth getting angry to survive. But people get just as angry because they punch the wrong key on a computer or because they say something on the telephone that causes them to lose a deal. People go berserk because their favorite sports team loses. The poison of anger destroys your body even if it's for good reason—no matter what the cause.

How many times a day can a person get angry? Once you get irritated, it becomes increasingly easy to become angry again. When you get angry enough, everyone becomes an enemy. Everyone seems to have a hidden agenda to cross you. Anger morphs into paranoia, so when you respond with ill intent you feel completely justified. The solution is to practice: ice to water, water to space.

Personal Practice Session 13

Take a moment to notice if you have anger inside you. As you start thinking about anger, rub against your liver (see p. 37 to find the location of the liver). Make yourself aware of the ways in which anger can also be a bodily experience. Anger is not only a mental thought or emotion. You may think about how someone lied to you or how you lost in a situation when you really wanted to win. If you have been in a big fight, you could think about the argument. If someone has wronged you, you could think about how that person crossed the line for the last time. There are a million reasons to get mad. What is frustrating you? Pick something and focus on it.

Begin dissolving from the top of your head. As you find a blockage, see if you can go to the energy behind, behind, behind. Is there any anger? Notice the energy behind the blockage. What is generating it? As a story comes up in your head to justify your anger, see if you can recognize how any story is rooted in the neutral quality of anger, the ability to take appropriate action. If you practice meditation a lot, you reach a point where you can release the ability to take action without going mad. If anger is sometimes necessary to break through a logjam in your own mind, you will more likely stop yourself in the middle and recognize anger for the purpose it serves. Slowly, over time, you start moving from needing to get angry to being able to use anger productively while leaving its potential poison behind.

Compassion, love and kindness help flip anger to its positive aspect. The force to create nurtures life and is the antidote to all negativity. Compassion and love are the only antidotes to anger and hatred. Anger and hatred sit right next to each other, but hatred is more extreme. Look for this force to take action inside you. Make that an agen-

da: What is the agenda of anger? Over time, make your agenda about where the negative side of action lies within you. Next, make your agenda about where its positive and neutral sides reside within you. Then, when you encounter any situation requiring you to take action, you can unleash the power to do so in a positive way. Let go of the power to do and let it move toward compassion, kindness and generosity. Use that natural force inside you to do good, to balance situations that are unbalanced. The power to do will express itself. It may manifest as destruction or creation—this is the nature of the beast.

Denial Is Anger's Partner

Denial follows anger because when you are so angry, you don't want to recognize what you are doing. You throw up justifications. It makes you like steel. You feel secure in your destructive capacity. People cannot control everything that happens in life. They are continuously faced with an essential choice of moving between the two poles of the continuum—either towards negativity or towards positivity—although most people naturally gravitate somewhere in the middle. My teacher Liu said you can be compassionate toward a situation or you can hate it. Ultimately the desire to hold onto face, power or control leads to anger because you can never get everything you want exactly the way you want it. You cease being human and connecting with other people. That is the beginning of the process of demonization. You cannot consider another human being as less than a human being, unless you feel anger toward that person. It's just not possible.

You need to have the power to do; otherwise, you cannot take your next breath or formulate a thought. Every action requires power, but combine that need with anger and the potential for frustration, and people will seek to control others and situations. Anger becomes the power to let our egos expand as far as humanly possible. Many of the most powerful people in ancient Chinese society were Taoists.

They were the equivalent of our governors, secretaries of state and generals in the Pentagon. At a certain point, these Taoists recognized that power over others and the desire for power to control the universe was empty. Taking action to control everything was empty and meaningless.

The only true power worth pursuing is that which leads to balance and compassion, which anger and frustration defeat. This incredible wisdom from the ancient world has not changed for more than 2,000 years. In the Taoist tradition, one of the primary practices is to learn to give up the sense of power that seeks to control. By releasing the need for control, you simultaneously let go of anger. In the pursuit of power, there is no freedom, love, compassion or kindness to be found at the end of the road.

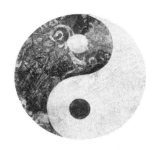

CHAPTER 14
Fear as an Agenda

Fear is a major part of the human condition and we need to be honest with ourselves about it. Something inside you wants to know the future. Are there any cultures in which astrology or scientific charts and graphs predicting the future don't draw a seriously big crowd? To the best of my knowledge, there aren't any. People fear that a given object, idea, feeling or being is not going to exist any longer. They want it to exist whether it's true or not. Eventually, the fear of loss begins to dominate and weakens the kidneys. The energy of all the internal organs is connected, so the other organs start spewing out their own emotions.

Our reptilian brain has fears that are evolutionary memories dating back to when we climbed out of the slime. In the modern world, people feel they have to fight for their ideas because they are considered important and real; we identify with our ideals. People activate both anger and fear when others don't acknowledge or validate their ideas. Because they identify with their ideals, threats upon their beliefs feel no different than the threats upon their very existence. People are more afraid of the idea of not existing than of their actual physical death. We have now moved from concrete situations to abstract thoughts. You can be fearful in 10,000 ways, but ultimately it's the inability to simply let go that brings about fear.

Confronting the Fear of Not Existing

One fundamental fear is the fear that you are not going to exist.[1] It's not really the fear of death or the physical act of dying that bothers people. They either make their peace with the idea that they are going to die or they don't. You may be afraid of death if someone close to you has passed away. You don't want it to happen to you. If you look behind the fear of death, you will notice that it's really about being afraid of not existing. Now, most people think they exist: "I'm me. Who else am I going to be?" And yet many meditative traditions assert that if you really start looking at who you actually are, you'll be hard-pressed to find anything.

From the age of six to twelve, I practiced what Indians call the Avida Vedanta, which was taught by a well-known man, Ramana Maharshi. Years later, I ended up going to his place in India and walked around the mountains he loved. He talked about going to the razor's edge—the edge between being spiritually awake and being asleep. It's difficult to find and even harder to stay with. Maharshi's basic method, at a very simple level, addresses the same question as Buddhism and Taoism: Do you really think you exist? In Sanskrit, it is called *neti neti*, meaning "neither this, nor that." Think of anything you identify with—your car, let's say. Okay. So, if your car weren't there, would you still be here? Yes. Similarly, you say you are this emotion or that: You are someone who hates; you are someone who loves. Maybe you identify with having accomplished this or that. Well, if you hadn't done this or that—you didn't hate and you didn't love—would you still be here? The only answer you can come up with is *yes*. If you follow this line of thought further, you realize that all the things you thought existed are not actually real. There's something else very hard to define. The reason why most people don't arrive at this point is that they think death is the root of fear. Yet it's not the fear of physical death—it's the fear of not existing.

People hold on to the belief that "I am something," and fill in the blank. Their ego derives from an identity, so they have to defend

[1] See the author's book, *Relaxing into Your Being*.

and expand it. I am my suffering, my hedonism, my successes, my failures. So when a human being thinks that whatever they fixate on is going to disappear, immense fear arises. Take the fear of losing your job and health insurance. In truth, you have no way of knowing if a better job with health insurance is going to come along. Further, if you fear the loss of job security yet you know that your job is killing you, what are you really afraid of? That you will lose your pain and suffering? That you will lose something that has become a habit? There are millions and millions of reasons to be fearful.

When you are afraid, your kidneys weaken. According to Chinese medicine, your kidneys are the source of your life force. They kick off the energetic cycle that makes your internal organs strong or weak. So whenever people become very fearful, it feels as though the life is leaving them, and this is why they think they fear death. You have to take one step back and look at why your kidneys were weakened in the first place. Fear may make people become passive-aggressive. Sublimated fear can turn to anger. Fear twisted in another way creates greed, power and egomaniacs. The list goes on. There is no end to it.

Even though people fear pain, they often won't let it go. People will often hold on to their suffering more than they will hold on to any pleasure. It is actually easier to give up pleasure than it is to give up pain. Pain and suffering are much more addictive than pleasure. Pain captivates people. Turn on the news and you will see for yourself that 70 percent of the stories are about pain and suffering. We are intrinsically attracted to fear and suffering as part of the human condition.

> *People will often hold on to their suffering more than they will hold on to any pleasure.*

Dissolving Fear as an Agenda

When you start dissolving without a specific agenda, from the top of your head to the bottom of your belly, you may not actually tap into an immediately recognizable vein of fear in your emotions. You may tap into an anger vein or a greed vein, which is fine. However, if you know you want to work on a specific agenda, then allow your mind to become magnetized toward fear and begin contemplating it. For the next few minutes, focus on the emotion of fear as you scan downward. You may think about losing all of your money in the stock market or being unable to pay your rent or mortgage. If you are worried about becoming sick, you could think about illness. If you have wronged someone, you could think about that person never forgiving you. There are a million fears to be had. What are your fears? Pick one.

You can go about it in two ways. You can just keep on thinking about fear in general, or you can think about a particular kind of fear that you have—formulate an agenda. It doesn't much matter because if your mind focuses on fear, your energy will start moving toward where it lives inside you. When you truly become free inside, you will no longer have fear. You may have realistic concerns about particular situations, but you won't have generalized fear. You will have accepted that the future is unknowable. Fear makes you think you know the future and so you expect negative consequences if something that you would like to exist is not going to exist. I don't know what it is that you want to exist, but I know it comes from fear.

When you start thinking about fear, press against your back where your kidneys are located. Make yourself aware of the ways in which fear can also be a bodily experience. Fear is not only a mental thought or emotion. Sit down and think about fear for a few minutes before you start meditating. Think about what exactly frightens you. After 10 minutes, let your mind completely relax. Let everything go out of your mind and just sit there and wait. At some point you will get a very light sense of fear, or at least some sense of stirring inside. Start from the top of your head and dissolve down to the bottom of your belly.

As you continue dissolving down from the top of your head, you are always feeling for the energy that is behind whatever comes into your awareness. Thoughts will come into your awareness and you will start talking to yourself. It's very important that you don't try to edit the thoughts. Stay with and dissolve the energy behind them. Suddenly you can find yourself going into an entirely different space of your inner world than where you have ever been before. Let whatever thoughts, whatever conversations you are having in your head—the monkey mind jumping from tree to tree—come up, but keep aware of the energy behind these conversations. Keep dissolving and staying focused on the energy behind the fear you are feeling.

 ## Author-guided Practice Session 14

Stop letting fear paralyze you: see p. 167.

Stop letting fear paralyze you: see p. 167.

Spacing Out and Internal Fog

Every once in a while, you are bound to get carried away with day-dreaming when you are working with the energy of fear. You start going down a path and find yourself spaced out because you are no longer focused on the energy that is behind it but instead have become absorbed in your internal conversation. You blink and come back, thinking, "Where am I? What's going on?" If you are still pretty close to the same spot in your body that you were dissolving, just feel for that quality of energy and keep tracking it back to its source. Continuously keep dissolving, ice to water, and you will go deeper and deeper inside yourself with the intent of releasing into space.

You are very actively waiting for the fear to release, staying com-pletely aware. It's like a cat waiting for a mouse. The cat has to stay with the mouse, waiting very quietly, because when the mouse moves to run down the hole, the cat has to be ready. When the emptiness opens up inside you, everything releases. If you space out, it's as if the cat blinks or goes to sleep. So when the mouse runs away, he can't catch up to it. Active waiting is something most of us aren't used to doing. We are part of an extremely yang culture that teaches us to push and strain. Nevertheless, just be patient and wait until every-thing softens and opens up. Active waiting makes your awareness become extremely clear. Your thoughts may change and stories will come up. Whatever the story is, stay with the energy behind it. Eventually, clarity will help you resolve the fear of the unknown—the fear of fear itself. Ice to water—release deeply and let go until at some point it all goes to space.

It's very important to recognize what happens if you space out when you are working with fear. You come back and you don't know where you left off. You almost feel as though cold water was thrown into your face when you were in a deep sleep. If you find yourself in this situation and you can't go back to the place you left off—you feel the energy there—go back to the top of your head again and let your mind just focus on fear. If you completely disconnect from wherever the thread was leading you inside, the connection has been broken and you need to start all over again from the top of your head.

Unexpressed Fear

Sometimes fear will turn into other things. It's quite normal for unexpressed fear to become anger. If you have thoughts of anger, keep moving through that energy to where fear is connected. Continue dissolving the energy behind what is generating your ideas. You may find yourself drifting back to your past, when you were small or found yourself in certain difficult circumstances that created fear. You may even go back to a time when everything was going well, yet you had this dreaded fear that it wasn't going to last. Always pay attention to the energy behind your thoughts and emotions and the energy behind that, going deeper and deeper toward your core.

Bodily Fear

As time goes on, you will also encounter and become aware of bodily fear. When a part of your body is diseased, the body has a natural fear mechanism to protect it. If you walked to the edge of a cliff and leaned over it, hopefully you would be afraid. Something inside of you becomes aware of real danger with consequences. Yet in modern society, we seem so sophisticated, and we have so many thoughts and 10,000 justifications about why we are afraid, that when we actually should have fear about a real circumstance, we don't. We become desensitized to real danger. Many people are numb. So they walk into the wrong neighborhood and into the wrong situation, even when everything inside them says they shouldn't be there. They think that they understand what is going on and keep on going. What is it inside of you that urges you to leave? Start to recognize if your body is signaling real fear. Very often, with little information or from pure intuition, we know that we should be concerned about something. Learn to recognize genuine fear.

The Three Aspects of Fear

As you go further into your fear, you may encounter different states. Every emotion has three sides to it: the negative side, from which all the problems arise; a neutral side, which serves a practical function for staying alive; and, finally, a positive side. In the process of dissolving through all your blockages, you may run into any one of these three aspects and it's useful to recognize them. Most people don't recognize the neutral and positive value of fear. The negative aspect of fear is terror and paralysis. The useful aspect is that it makes you aware. If you are standing in front of a car that is moving toward you at 100 miles an hour, you need to jump out of the way. Awareness is necessary, with it you have the ability to act.

All the spiritual traditions say that, on the other side of death, your inner body becomes more awake. The *Tao Te Ching* has a wonderful phrase that says, "No animal can gore him, death cannot touch him." It means that the person has moved beyond fear. It doesn't refer to a real rhinoceros, which could kill most anybody. Lao Tse is referring to the fear of not existing, of being unwilling to engage fully with life. While you are fearful, you are not fully alive. You are always hedging your bets.

You may realize that fear is dominating your life and that you would like the fear to cease. In the next blockage you encounter, see if fear shows itself. See if the root of the fear reveals itself. Follow the little fear to the bigger fear to the giant fear until finally you realize that all fear is the same. There are not a million different kinds of fear. There is either freedom or there is fear. It is perfectly fine to be afraid when you are on the edge of a cliff, but realize that it is really an awareness of what can happen. It's not the fear of an idea you have of what can happen. Fear is meant to motivate you to take an action of some kind. If you let fear overwhelm you, it can be paralyzing or cause you to act in ways that bring more harm. On the flip side, if you have no fear, you might just walk right over the edge of that cliff. So find the balance point where fear neither ceases to serve its function nor causes so much unnecessary anxiety that it interferes with your life choices.

The Root of All Fear

In the midst of the Great Depression, when times were hard and many people had little to eat, the president of the United States, Franklin Delano Roosevelt, himself a

> *After you have worked through your more superficial fears, you come to the ultimate fear agenda: I no longer wish to be afraid of being fully alive and awake.*

cripple from polio, made the famous declaration: "There is nothing to fear but fear itself." Fear diminishes our life force. If you are afraid of death, you can never make peace with it. Fear presents itself in many forms, but the root of all fear is the thought that something exists and that it might not continue to exist. After you have worked through your more superficial fears, you come to the ultimate fear agenda: I no longer wish to be afraid of being fully alive and awake. You must overcome fear to be awake and have peace of mind. Let it serve its purpose to keep you aware and prevent you from taking dangerous or unmitigated risks, but you don't have to let fear dominate your life.

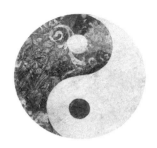

CHAPTER 15
Pain as an Agenda

In some way or another, pain follows us every day. Some people experience more, some less. Pain can come from many different directions. Physical pain is a fact of life for many. Studies show that meditation helps with managing physical pain. In many ways, however, emotional pain is even worse to live through and mental pain of the mind churning can be worse still. The most horrible is existential pain or angst, the vague sense of being unresolved and living a life that lacks meaning.

Physical Pain

The vast majority of pain is just sensation. We might call it pain because we can't enter into it, yet we experience these massive sensations. Learning to dissolve and let go of a sensation can be immensely valuable to reducing your experience of pain. Dissolving may work when medications don't.

I've experienced a lot of pain in my life, a fact that doesn't make me terribly unique. When I was twenty-three, I suffered from a severe case of hepatitis. Both people on either side of me died. I was told that I would die too. At the edge of death, I was luckily able to survive because, using tai chi, I learned how to open the energy channels of my body and this skill kept me from ticking over to the other side.[1] As a martial artist, I had broken bones before, but that was nothing compared to the pain of opening up my blocked channels while I was suffering from an extremely virulent case of hepatitis. According to Chinese medicine, blocked chi causes pain and disease whereas unblocked chi does not cause pain and disease. So to the extent that your chi is blocked and not flowing, you proportionally feel pain and become diseased. Pain and diseases come about along a continuum. Conversely, when your chi is unblocked you neither get sick nor do you feel pain. From personal experience, I have found that you can reduce many severe kinds of pain dramatically if you know what to do. You can also sit and dissolve the pain of "I" or "you."

Besides dissolving my body in general, I used a specific method for my spine after I broke my back in a car accident. Sitting, I would dissolve and let go—ice to water, water to gas. You start at the base of your head where your spine meets your skull, also known as the occipital junction or atlas axis, which happens to be the site of the most common chiropractic adjustment. You start here and dissolve—ice to water, water to gas—and trace down your spine inch by inch, using all the instructions described in the previous chapters about locating any of the four conditions. Sometimes it would take me three, four or five hours to dissolve from the top of my neck down to the bottom of my tailbone. I experienced massive sensations that I had chosen to interpret as pain. Sometimes I was screaming the whole time. At the very least, self-pity would paralyze me. I was angry at being alive because obviously I should have been dead. I was fearful for what the next day was going to be like when the pain got worse. When these emotions arose, I changed ice to water, water to space to better resolve them.

I was frustrated because after having dissolved and gone through the emotions hundreds of times I expected the process to be finished, but it wasn't. All I had was the chance, one day at a time, to go

---

[1] See the author's book, *Tai Chi: Health for Life*, Chapter 3, to learn some of the techniques he used.

from being half alive to being fully alive. There were no guarantees that my situation was ever going to get better. And still I would dissolve through it. The sensations would become incredibly powerful at times. It was electric, sometimes burning, and I did a lot of swearing. But that was not the worst of it.

Most people would not consider that having their backs smashed to pieces could be one of the better things to happen to them in life, but I do. Something happened for me. While I was working with the physical pain, dissolving each vertebra, I went deeper and started becoming acutely aware of how my spinal injury affected every energy channel in my body. If you are really hurt, you have the chance to discover where all the pain is in your channels and all the ways in which they are blocked. Then you have the opportunity to release, dissolve and resolve these blockages.

When those channels clear, a much deeper level of your body is no longer in pain. Clarity arises and you start seeing many things you have done in your life for what they are, without sugarcoating or drama. You don't think about how wonderful or terrible a person you were. You just start seeing life for what it is and freeing yourself from your stories. You begin to accept that you are not a god who shouldn't feel pain, but a human being with a fragile body, mind and energy system. You must accept your humanity.

 ## Author-guided Practice Session 15

Dissolve your physical pain: see p. 167.

Becoming a Mature Human Being

During this period, my teacher Liu told me a story about when he was a young man and wanted to be a hero. When he began studying Buddhism and Taoism, he realized that wanting to be a hero was an incredible weight to carry, a burden that no human being should have to suffer. So, just as Liu did, I decided that being human was quite enough. I didn't need to be the greatest man or hero, and I didn't have to live up to any image that had nothing to do with me. Liu also said that when you are going through a temporary period of pain, there's no need to be a hero. Bravery is okay. Perseverance is okay, but you don't need to be more than human.

As time went on, Liu explained to me that the Taoists consider becoming a mature human being one of the greatest goals any person can attain. Most people, because they try to be more than human, never reach their humanity. So I worked through the pain and at a certain point I started feeling how all of my emotions existed within those channels. Then I started feeling the pain of my emotions. I felt the pain of my anger, fear, greed, pride, jealousy, hopes and expectations, and slowly but surely it started becoming very obvious that all of these things were only in my mind. When I released the pain in my emotions, sometimes the bodily pain would also cease for three or four days. I have to say that my ability to handle emotional pain was greater than my ability to handle that level of physical pain.

Maybe you have some pain now. Some people have minor pains, others have severe pains. There are bumps and

> *Most people, because they try to be more than human, never reach their humanity.*

bruises and there are major accidents and illnesses. Many diseases can make you feel so much pain and yet the more you notice, the more you will see that it's all just about sensations. The pain in your body, the pain in your energy channels and the pain of your emotions are all sensations. Sometimes you want to jump out of your skin, but go into the sensation. Don't try to run away from it or shut it off. In the Taoist tradition, it is said that to fight a dragon you should jump right into its throat when it opens its mouth to breathe fire or bite you, and you should either pull its tongue or teeth out. So go into the pain without fear. Even if you are afraid, just keep going. Ice to water, water to space.

Pain is interesting because it has many shades and textures. As you release each layer, eventually a great area inside you opens and there is a clarity and freedom from the burden on your soul. If the release is incredibly strong, you will feel freedom—as if you have just been taken off a torture table. For those who are afflicted with chronic pain, everything settles down, but the process will start all over again. There is no easy solution; all you might be able to do is lessen the pain. Continuing to go through the layers is very important. After you have had some giant release from pain, you will notice the pain again, or some other blockage that leads you to the energy behind, behind, behind.

The Pain of Thought

The pain of thinking that never stops is not purely emotional, although such pain can make you feel sad, tortured or miserable. It's the kind of pain Vincent van Gogh felt trying to paint the perfect sunflowers. Some thoughts cannot be resolved and they have no peace. At the moment you come to a resolution, another thought is created and springs up to rip you apart again. You have to actually go to the root of what is driving those thoughts in the first place and release them. Even the great genius Sir Isaac Newton went through a period in his life where he got so obsessed with his thinking and calculations that he had a complete nervous breakdown. He had to stop working for months and was on bed rest. Thoughts can wear us down and eventually burn us out just as easily as they can bring great joy. There is pleasure in learning and acquiring knowledge that goes beyond anything the physical body can do. It isn't better, just different. And yet, if thoughts go too far, they can tear us apart as much as a poison ravages our system because, below where you think, below the place from which conscious thoughts originate, is the great unconscious mind. It's the place from which your thoughts arise. If there is no peace your thoughts can drive you to mental pain and anguish, destroying all peace in your life.

Today in the fast-paced computer age, we can easily burn out from incredibly intense mental work. The nervous system cannot sustain it. A place exists before a thought comes into our heads. You must find this place and put your intent there to dissolve and resolve what is there if you are ever to find mental peace.

Author-guided Practice Session 16

Dissolve the pain of thinking: see p. 167.

Emotional Pain

Emotional pain is very deep. When emotional pain is not released and instead sits and festers, it has a nasty habit of recreating itself again and again. Families often carry emotional pain from one generation to the other, like a virus or sickness.

The difficulty with emotional pain is that most people don't realize that they're going through it. So they may lash out at others or take it out on themselves. Having taught tai chi to inmates in prisons, I found that a huge proportion of the people who committed the worst crimes frequently had been beaten and ill-treated by their parents or other caretakers. These are extreme cases; yet emotional pain binds everyone. If it isn't released, like a grain of sand that gets stuck inside an oyster shell, the next pain wraps around the previous one until eventually you have a pearl. It's that pearl of poison that drives people crazy. Pain drives people mad. Releasing ice to water, water to space can be done immediately when something painful happens to you.

If you recognize any of these qualities of emotional pain within yourself, you can make it an agenda to release them. After preparing yourself, go back to the top of your head. As you dissolve downwards, release the root of your pain so that, for example, you don't have to drink, keep apologizing or live a half-life anymore. Unresolved pain doesn't go away. It's like acid that eats up your insides. Pain can come from many sources. You may have flunked out of school; someone may have cheated you; you may have suffered the pain of betrayal or being hated. If great pain comes upon you for whatever reason, simply have the courage to acknowledge what has happened and release it. Ice to water, water to space. If you focus, you can let it go. When you let go, you become free. When you become free, you don't have to spread pain to the next person. Instead, the space where balance and compassion arises will open up inside you.

 ## Author-guided Practice Session 17

Dissolve your emotions: see p. 167.

Dissolve your emotions: see p. 167.

Loss of a Loved One

For a moment, consider if you are still grieving for anyone who has passed away. The day before my teacher Liu died, he finished teaching me the final piece of what I had been studying with him in China for several years. From my point of view, what he did was fairly magical. The next morning I walked down the street towards his house. As always, I was practicing martial arts as I walked. The locals knew my teacher was a great martial arts master, so they were used to seeing me do this move or that with the look of, "Oh, there goes that foreigner again!" This morning though they started laughing at me. Someone asked me what I was doing, but I could not figure out what they were talking about. Then I walked into Liu's house and there he was, laid out dead on his bed. Yesterday was full of promise of what was to come, but today he had chosen to die about an hour before I arrived. I felt such immense grief and loss that I believed that nothing I did, said or thought mattered.

In time I dissolved, ice to water, water to space. At times I would be very tearful, at times I would be sullen, at times I would just be in shock. Eventually, the grief passed.

My grandfather, who raised me, was an extremely strong, silent type. Getting him to talk about the past and what happened to him in the old country, Greece, was about as easy as robbing Fort Knox. For my whole life, I wanted to know his story and the history of my family. Nothing. There was no way he would talk about it, although I longed for him to share our family's history with me. Finally, when I went to see him before he passed away, I looked him right in the eye and made it clear that I really needed to know about his past since I didn't know how much longer he was going to be around. For the first time in his life, he started talking about how he left Greece, how his high-society family wanted him to become a monk, how he was the youngest member of his family, how he managed to get out of the country and how the Nazis killed all the members of his family who remained in Greece. The point is that I made peace with him. If I had never had that conversation with him, this never would have happened. If I had not become resolved with my grandfather in this way, I think it would have bothered me for many years, maybe to the end of my life.

I have taken many of my students through meditation so they could resolve what happened with somebody who died since they didn't get the resolution they needed while that person was alive. Some people die suddenly, regardless of age or health. If you love and care about somebody—or even if you hate or have any other kind of powerful connection with somebody—you must release the energy between you and that person. Ice to water, water to space. Children need to release their parents so that their parents are free to live in peace. When children stand near a dying parent and don't want to let go, it burdens that parent immensely. It does not help them pass. Likewise, sometimes parents have to watch children die and there's nothing they can do about it. You have to do whatever is necessary—take days, weeks or months out of your life—and release that person. You cannot sacrifice the living for the dead. This is a very basic philosophy or religious practice that helps the human condition. Unless you release someone from the depths of your mind, the depths of your spirit, that person lives inside you. Depending on the degree to which they live inside you, they may tear you apart and steal your life. You cannot live your life. The joy you could have does not emerge because they are somewhere in the background siphoning it off.

> *You cannot sacrifice the living for the dead.*

In Taoism, one of the oldest meditative traditions on earth, it is considered very important when someone dies that you sit and dissolve him or her until you release that person. Taoists assert that it is essential for the soul to make its onward journey as smoothly and cleanly as possible. The person cannot be set free while you are holding on to them tightly. So if you care about someone, set them free. If you care about yourself, set yourself free. The regrets or grief no longer matter. Breathe in and breathe out—grief affects the lungs. Let go. Ice to water, water to space.

 ## Author-guided Practice Session 18

Dissolve your grief: see p. 167.

Dissolve your grief: see p. 167.

Other Kinds of Loss

You have to release that which binds you, so take the time to be free of your relationships, whether you break up with a boyfriend, girlfriend, husband, wife or business partner; have a falling out with a family member; a loved one moves to the other side of the world; or you wish to stop hating someone or hating yourself. Ice to water, water to space. Keep meditating.

Dissolving Your Pain

What kind of pain do you have? How many layers of pain do you have? There's a clarity that comes with awakening the psychic energy body—whether it's called illumination, such as in the contemplative traditions of Christianity, or enlightenment as it's called in the East. Everybody can recognize that they have a body and everyone, if they make the effort to look, can recognize a more subtle layer of energy in their body. Everyone can recognize that they have emotions and everyone can recognize that they think. All four of these elements can generate tremendous pain. Dissolving can release you from it. So although you may start with a sense of a particular pain, you may find yourself noticing how all pain is connected. Pain that is deep within your body has the power to numb you. Releasing pain makes you more sensitive and alive. Becoming fully alive is a major focus of meditation. Release, dissolve and resolve any sensations of whatever kind that might even remotely relate to any one of the four conditions. Ice to water, water to space.

Pain can be a great teacher. It would be absolutely wonderful if human beings did not have to learn and grow through pain and suffering. Unfortunately, it does seem to be that way. Yet if you release the source of the pain and suffering within you, it will be gone. With it, much freedom and joy—the natural state of human beings—can emerge. Pain blocks happiness and freedom—it makes them unrecognizable. Humor and laughter, as well as the ability to open up and connect so that we can see the absurdity of everything inside ourselves, are all part of sharing our humanity with others. Pain, denial, anger and frustration will seek to destroy these natural human qualities. Release pain and discover the joy in life. Ice to water, water to space.

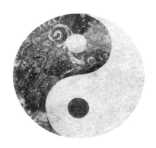

CHAPTER 16
Love and Compassion

Meditation Is a Circular Process

Everything in meditation, like emptiness, is circular. It has no beginning. It has no end. Within your inner world, everything flows from one part to the other. Every emotion and every thought you have in your life is a part of a cycle. The greatest scientists in the world, who think some of the most intelligent thoughts, can keep going around in circles, with each rotation going to a deeper place with greater implications. The human condition is filled with constant repeating activities, each one giving us the opportunity to remain foolish or become wise. Every breath you take is a circle. Every inhale is followed by an exhale and another inhale.

So thinking about a finite goal may be fine for the external world, but real life continues, deepens and moves from one thing to the next to the next. It never stops; it never completes itself. Even at the time of a person's death, another cycle begins.

Meditation takes you deeper into your inner world, deeper into the place where inner peace and joy are to be found. You cannot think of it as attaining a final goal or "been there, done that." If you applied this strategy to breathing, you would die. Likewise, if your world does not continuously evolve and grow, you will die, slowly but surely. However, if the cycle continues and evolves, slowly but surely you become more alive. I've written in my books many times that my teacher Liu said, "You become what you practice." If you practice that which creates more vital life-force energy, you will naturally wake up and become more alive.

The Greatest Gift You Can Give Yourself

We all have the ability to give gifts both to ourselves and to others. The gift of what is inside of you—discovering the depth of your inner world—is the greatest gift you can give yourself. The one thing that you live with every second of your life is the world inside you, the depth of your spirit. It's as close to permanence as anything will be in this life, so give yourself the gift of waking up. Everything else is unimportant by comparison.

The ancient Chinese had a proverb: First learn to rule yourself, know your inner world. Then rule your family; try to keep it together even under difficult circumstances. Then rule the world. They didn't talk about ruling the world and then ruling themselves. They first dealt with what was inside themselves in a pragmatic, intelligent, compassionate and loving way. Only then could they show compassion towards those who were closest to them and, eventually, extend that compassion to strangers.

Opening to Your Soul

Within the Taoist tradition, as well as in many other ancient traditions, love, compassion, genuine kindness and generosity play major roles for several very important reasons. There are many forms of negativity in the world, ranging from negative physical states to emotional states to mental states. The one antidote to the strongest forms of negativity is love and compassion. More hate will not resolve hate. More greed will not resolve greed. If your greed is to be a millionaire, becoming a billionaire will not satisfy your greed. But love, compassion and the genuine kindness coming from a place that asks for nothing in return will further love, compassion and genuine kindness. Love and compassion will open human beings to their souls.

Some people will claim that love and compassion are really self-serving and manipulative; that you expect reciprocity at some level.

Genuine love and kindness does not ask for anything in return.

While it's true that you can use what appears on the surface to be love or compassion to indebt or burden someone, that's not genuine love; it's a bargain. It's the "I love you, therefore you must love me" syndrome. It's the same as "I love you, therefore you must do what I want." It's a negotiation rather than love. Genuine love and kindness does not ask for anything in return.

 ## Author-guided Practice Session 19

Amplify your life force and open to love and compassion: see p. 167.

see p. 167.

Cultivate Compassion

Cultivating compassion in itself is not difficult. But many of us fall short of acting out the ideal of compassion because events happen and people do things that activate what is unresolved in us—physical, energetic, emotional, mental, psychic or karmic blockages. In effect, we are rendered incapable of acting in accordance with what we know to be right. For example, very few smokers don't know that cigarettes cause serious illnesses, such as emphysema and lung cancer, which result in tens of thousands of deaths every year. Yet they make the decision several times a day to smoke, even when they say they wish they wouldn't. Why? They have not gone to the root of what is causing the smoking in the first place. They have not yet released the blockage underlying the symptom—and the self-hatred associated with not following their ideals can exacerbate the symptoms.

Taoists believe that any wise human being will go towards compassion. You have to become present to understand and apply your intent to make positive change. Ultimately, the only way the universe will open itself to someone—and the only way the human heart will truly open—is through compassion, through love. This includes self-love. We so often get used to acting from a place of conditional love, rather than true, open love. If you cannot open up to yourself, you cannot open up to another human being. You love because you are loved. Your heart opens of its own accord. There was no one Jesus Christ hated. There was no one Buddha hated. There was no one Lao Tse hated. They had compassion. They had love for whomever they met. I'm sure they chose not to spend time with certain people, but they felt and showed compassion for everyone just the same.

The World May Go Crazy, but You Don't Have To

The whole world may seem to go crazy, but individual human beings don't have to if enough compassion and love opens up within them. Taoists say that you first seek to become balanced so you can take on whatever it is you want to do. Only then do you seek wisdom, which will set the stage for your natural courage to flow and engage in compassion. To become balanced, you have to let go. Dissolve and let go.

APPENDIX 1:
Taoist Meditation for Health

Every Body Is Different

Humans have different levels of tolerance to stress and pressure. Some lead completely dissolute lifestyles and live long, healthy lives; others live as purely as possible and have short, miserable ones. The difference lies primarily in the amount of energy they were born with and often in the strength of their nervous systems.

From the Chinese point of view, the capacity to bear stress is a function of the strength of the nerves. When the stress level surpasses the central nervous system's coping ability, the nerves begin to break down, which results in all sorts of physical, emotional and mental disturbances, and which can eventually lead to organ malfunction. Since people's nervous systems differ in strength, it is important that practices account for these differences.

Chi Travels through the Nerves

Every message from the brain to the body, and vice versa, goes through the central nervous system. When practicing directly manipulates the central nervous system, three precautions must be taken. First, the practice must be done within the proper limits or the nerves can be damaged. Second, the new pathways must lead to health and well-being, not illness. Finally, the body must have enough time to balance out all these new inputs, so that the signal is not scrambled. Going too fast may cause problems for both the mind and body; it may also lead to imagining that things are happening when they are not.

Is the Dissolving Process Working for Me?

The best guidepost is a simple before-and-after comparison. Where were you internally after dissolving? Is the sting of any blockages you identified the same, less or different? Have you dissolved and gone past one more layer of your negative emotional onion and become aware of what is really underneath your initial reaction? After focusing for some days, weeks or months, are you moving toward resolution of a lifelong problem or at least finding that you can now cope better with it, without it tearing up your insides? Does the Dissolving process help you to reach equanimity with what used to be an irresolvable and highly charged set of feelings inside you? Are you beginning to change?

You can use agendas to target specific negative emotions or emotional patterns, dissolve them, and personally experience change. First, find something that perpetually gets your negative emotions going, reflexively. There are so many: a memory of a perceived wrong done to you, a political position you cannot abide, something you are immensely jealous of, something that makes you salivate with greed, a person or group you don't like, a deep regret, a painful memory that will not leave or an unresolved hangover from your relationship with your parents, lovers, friends or enemies. Second, focus on dissolving the obstacles that keep you from generating any positive state you may want to establish—for example, the ability to be tolerant, to love, to accept love and to live without fear.

Gradually, you will build enough experience to know internally whether dissolving has in fact occurred or whether you have only shifted the same piece of content from one place on your internal board to another without substantially changing anything. Of course, the more subtle the content you are working on, the greater your sensitivity must be to realistically discriminate between definable internal landmarks in this very subjective area. Conversely, the grosser or more violent the emotions you are dealing with, the easier it will be to gauge whether something is happening.

Energy Flow Follows Toxin Release

Keep in mind that in the early stages of practice, say the first few months, the body practice may release a tremendous amount of stored toxins, which can result in feelings of fatigue, discomfort or an unwillingness to continue practicing. Toxins are released through the sweat, urine and feces, and in the beginning, you may notice that your sweat smells unpleasant. This will pass and soon your sweat will be relatively odorless.

Cultivate Your Chi Slowly and Safely

All safe chi development practices are cumulative and progress slowly while developing powerful links with the brain. You are training your nerves how to convey messages between the mind and the chi clearly with sufficient insulation and resistance to avoid burnout. A strong nervous system allows messages to be delivered between the brain and the chi without conscious will or effort. Until the nerves have been developed, the will must be used to transmit messages. A baby first has to use tremendous willpower and concentration to crawl and walk until the appropriate nerve pathways are forged between the brain and the chi. Once those links are in place, you need not to think about walking—you simply walk. The development of chi must, by necessity, be slow and steady in order for it to stabilize.

Meditation for Stress Management

For people involved in high-stress jobs, it is important to understand how stress works, which is discussed in Chapter 2. Stress begins with overexcitement of the nervous system and then slowly works its way deep into the body. It begins as wet cement, so to speak, and when the stress is prolonged, the cement begins to harden. That is, the contraction and constriction of the nerves and organs starts to become permanent. The stress of the morning begins to harden around lunchtime. The stress accumulated after lunch will begin to set by evening or the end of the workday.

Five minutes spent identifying whether any of the four conditions are present and then breathing into those areas can prove to be of great value. In effect, you are wiping away the day's stress and keeping the metaphorical cement wet. Ten or 15 minutes at lunch can bring back the freshness of the morning. Practice after work can take away all the stress accumulated during the day—before the wet cement has a chance to dry.

Any practice above and beyond this initial stress release will increase your core energy reserves, which your body and mind use in times of crisis, emergency, or recovery from illness or accident. This core reserve of chi will also determine the quality of energy available later in your life.

Practicing Meditation and Use of Prescription Drugs

The prescription drugs of allopathic medicine, along with herbal or homeopathic remedies, are normally used to ameliorate some kind of disease. To the best of my knowledge, practicing Taoist meditation while taking any of these medicines is safe insofar as physiologically based problems are concerned.

Taoist meditation has been used for millennia to restore health or to enhance the medical procedures of massage, acupuncture, bone setting and the herbal remedies found in traditional Chinese medicine. This tradition continues in China today as hospitals apply tai chi, qigong and methods of meditation to a great variety of physical problems. In these hospitals, both traditional Chinese medicine and Western allopathic medicine, including drugs and surgery, complement each other and they are integrated to obtain maximum benefit for the patient.

The experience in China has been that the Water methods of meditation, being sufficiently gentle, are safe; however, there are cautions, such as in the case of drugs that can lower or raise blood pressure. To be certain, consult your physician.

Practicing Meditation and Use of Recreational Drugs

Taoists believe that recreational drugs dull clarity of mind and thereby retard or completely block progress toward the deeper levels of meditation. True, you can point to a large variety of cultures worldwide that have employed any number of mind-altering drugs to enter into psychic realms. Some of these drugs are integral parts of solid spiritual traditions, but are not part of the Water method of Taoism, which purely uses the five modes of practice (standing, moving, sitting, lying down and partner exercises) with no external support.

We live in a world where drug use, including alcohol and tobacco, is rampant. Many who use one drug or another also meditate. A Taoist would typically look at this reality and ponder the practical ramifications involved.

Many young people try recreational drugs to experience the "something more" they feel is inside themselves, but cannot access. The use of hallucinogens, for example, often gives the drug taker an expanded internal experience of the possibilities of the body-mind. Such mind-spirit expansions are potentially good, but exploring them with drugs may exact a terrible price. Drug-induced visions, moreover, are not even a remote shadow of what the spirit and consciousness have to offer a human being.

Once drug users learn, through Taoist meditation, to go inside and find the living spiritual root that dwells there—however slowly, since drugs will impede their progress—they just might reduce their intake or perhaps even stop using drugs altogether.

Medical Advice

All material provided in this text is offered for informational or educational purposes only and is not intended as a substitute for the advice of your physician, psychotherapist or other healthcare professional. If you have any physical or other symptoms, or any emotional, mental or medical condition, please consult your healthcare provider regarding whether or not the exercises in this book are appropriate for you.

APPENDIX 2:
Practice Sessions

Practice Sessions will improve your health and serve as a highly useful aid to grounding your mind, an indispensable quality necessary for any form of meditation. The big challenge in learning the preparatory phase of Taoist meditation is gaining the ability to have your mind become concentrated on what you are doing for an extended period of time without becoming distracted. These practices are immensely valuable for reducing stress and for building stamina.

Personal Practice Sessions

Thirteen Practice Sessions are integrated into the main text to help you understand the purpose of each exercise. You can either take a break to try some of the practices, or save them for later when you're not simultaneously engaged in an intellectual activity.

Don't be in a rush to move on to the next practice. Take your time and develop and integrate each new skill before moving on to learning the next one.

Author-guided Practice Sessions

Eventually you will have to lay down the book and spend some hours in your comfy chair or on a zafu. When you go inside, all you will encounter is yourself. All time and guidelines tend to fall by the wayside.

Many of Bruce Frantzis' students have used the companion meditation course (six-CD set) to this book, also entitled *Tao of Letting Go*, to help guide them through their practice sessions. You can choose to listen to a specific track repeatedly, just have one of the CDs on to get you started, or to work with a sequence of tracks.

Ancient Chinese Chanting

The tradition of Taoist meditation includes chanting liturgies in ancient Chinese to work with and change the energetic frequencies within a human being.

Frantzis trained as a Taoist priest in China, during which time he learned 3,000 ancient liturgies. He has used these powerfully effective chants since the 1980s to help his students relax their tension, energetic blockages, emotions and churning thoughts.

These chants are in effect the music of the spheres—ancient audio technology developed by the Taoists thousands of years ago for people to activate their eight energy bodies and weave them together. These liturgies can help you:

- Enhance your ability to breathe fully into your body

- Become present and experience Fourth Time

- Align your body to ensure uninhibited chi flow for optimal health

- Transform fear, rejection and depression into awareness, freedom and joy

- Deepen your meditation practice

- Relax into the Heart-Mind to allow love and compassion to flow freely.

You can listen to a sample liturgy at EnergyArts.com to help you become present, or use Frantzis' *Ancient Songs of the Tao* (three-CD set) of liturgies to help you while you practice.

All Personal Practice Sessions are stand-alone and do not require the use of the audio set in conjunction with the teaching.

Coordinate Your Personal and Guided Practice Sessions

The page numbers below correspond with references to the Author-guided Practice Sessions as follows:

	Author-guided Practice Session			*Tao of Letting Go* (6-CD set)		*Ancient Songs of the Tao* (3-CD set)	
#	Subject	Page	Disc	Track	Disk	Track
1	Breathing	31	1	6	1	8–21
			2	7	–	–
2	Moving the diaphragm	34	2	7	1	10–11
3	Alignments	49	1	8	2	1–8
4	Four conditions	63	2	1–6	–	–
5	Fist tightening	79	3	2	–	–
6	Fourth Time	91	3	5	2	13–14
7	Dissolve downwards	97	3	6	–	–
			6	6	–	–
8	Distraction	101	3	6	–	–
			6	4–5	–	–
9	Emotions and shock	105	3	7–8	3	All
10	Fog and depression	114	4	4–7	3	4–7
11	Agendas and expectations	119	4	1, 8–9	2	13–14
12	Anxiety	122	6	2	3	12–13
13	Anger and frustration	128	5	1	3	2–3
14	Fear	137	4	2	3	8–9
15	Physical pain	143	5	2	3	14–15
16	Pain of thought	145	5	3	3	14–15
17	Emotional pain	147	5	4	3	14–15
18	Grief	149	5	5–6	–	–
19	Love and compassion	153	6	1	3	16–17

APPENDIX 3:
Taoism: A Living Tradition

Many traditions based on ancient philosophies and religions have vibrantly continued into modern times. Because they manifest in our lives today, they are called living traditions. These include Christianity, Islam, Judaism, Buddhism, yoga and Taoism. The latter three have clear practices that concentrate on physical exercises and energy work.

Taoism is the least known of the living traditions. Although its main literary works—the *I Ching*, the writings of Chuang Tse, and the *Tao Te Ching* by Lao Tse—are well known and available in many translations, the practical methods and techniques of implementing Taoist philosophy in daily life are little documented in the West.

The Taoist lineages that Bruce Frantzis holds and teaches today are in the Water tradition of Taoism, which has received minimal exposure in the West. Part of his lineage empowers and directs him to bring practices based on that tradition to Westerners. He learned the Chinese language and became immersed in the traditions of China during his training there, which spanned a decade. This has enabled him to bridge the gap between Chinese culture and the West and to bring living Taoism to Westerners in a way that they can comprehend and learn.

While Frantzis studied with his main teacher, Grandmaster Liu Hung Chieh, texts were presented as: "This is what they say; this is what they mean; this is how to do them." Frantzis offers an unprecedented bridge to this pragmatic approach to spirituality; in fact, we are not aware of any other English or European language source for this style of teaching. It means that spirituality is not just an aspiration for which people strive in the dark—"in a mirror, darkly"—to quote St. Paul, but it can become a genuine, accomplishable reality.

The Frantzis Energy Arts System

Drawing on sixteen years of training in Asia, Bruce Frantzis has developed a practical, comprehensive system of programs that can enable people of all ages and fitness levels to increase their core energy and attain vibrant health.

The Frantzis Energy Arts® system includes six primary qigong courses that, together with the Longevity Breathing® program, progressively and safely incorporate all the aspects of neigong—the original chi cultivation (qigong) system in China invented by the Taoists. Although the qigong techniques are very old, Frantzis' system of teaching them is unique. This method is specifically tailored to Westerners and the needs of modern life.

Core Qigong Practices

The core practices consist of:

- Longevity Breathing®
- Dragon and Tiger Medical Qigong
- Opening the Energy Gates of Your Body™ Qigong
- Marriage of Heaven and Earth™ Qigong
- Bend the Bow™ Spinal Qigong
- Spiraling Energy Body™ Qigong
- Gods Playing in the Clouds™ Qigong

The core qigong programs were deliberately chosen because they are among the oldest, most effective, and most treasured of Taoist energy practices. They are ideal for progressively incorporating the major components of neigong in a manner that is comprehensible to Westerners. These practices give students the foundation for clearly and systematically learning and advancing their practice in Taoist energy arts.

Longevity Breathing Program

This program teaches authentic Taoist breathing in systematic stages. Breathing with the whole body has been used for millennia to enhance the ability to dissolve and release energy blockages in the mind-body, enhancing well-being and spiritual awareness. Incorporating these breathing techniques into any other Taoist energy practice will help bring out its full potential.

Dragon and Tiger Medical Qigong

This is one of the most direct and accessible low-impact qigong healing methods that China has produced. This 1,500-year-old form of medical qigong affects the human body in a manner similar to acupuncture. Its seven simple movements can be done by virtually anyone, whatever their age or state of health.

Opening the Energy Gates of Your Body Qigong

This program introduces 3,000-year-old qigong techniques that are fundamental to advancing any energy arts practice. Core exercises teach you basic body alignments and how to increase your internal awareness of chi in your body and dissolve blocked chi.

Marriage of Heaven and Earth Qigong

This qigong incorporates techniques widely used in China to help heal back, neck, spine and joint problems. It is especially effective for helping to mitigate repetitive stress injury and carpal tunnel problems. This program teaches some important neigong components, including openings and closings (pulsing), more complex breathing techniques and methods for moving chi through the energy channels of the body.

Bend the Bow Spinal Qigong

Bend the Bow Spinal Qigong continues the work of strengthening and regenerating the spine that is learned in Marriage of Heaven and Earth qigong. This program incorporates neigong components for awakening and controlling the energies of the spine.

Spiraling Energy Body Qigong

This advanced program teaches you to dramatically raise your energy level and to master how energy moves in circles and spirals throughout your body. It incorporates neigong components for: directing the upward flow of energy; projecting chi along the body's spiraling pathways; delivering or projecting energy at will to or from any part of the body; and activating the body's left, right, and central channels, and the microcosmic orbit.

Gods Playing in the Clouds Qigong

Gods Playing in the Clouds incorporates some of the oldest, most powerful Taoist rejuvenation techniques. This program amplifies all the physical, breathing and energetic components taught in earlier qigong programs. Gods completes the process of integrating all sixteen components of neigong. It is also the final stage of learning to strengthen and balance the energies of your three tantiens (the primary centers in the human body where chi collects, disperses and recirculates), central energy channel and spine. Gods serves as a spiritual bridge to Taoist meditation.

Tai Chi and Ba Gua as Health Arts

Tai chi and ba gua practiced as health arts intensify the benefits of the core qigong practices.

Most Westerners learn tai chi purely as a health exercise rather than as a martial art. As with all qigong programs, tai chi relaxes and regulates the central nervous system, releasing physical and emotional stress, and promoting mental and emotional well-being. Tai chi's gentle, nonjarring movements are ideal for people of any age and body type and can give the practitioner a high degree of relaxation, balance and physical coordination.

Even more ancient than tai chi, the Circle Walking techniques of ba gua were developed over 4,000 years ago in Taoist monasteries as a health and meditation art. The techniques open up the potential of the mind to achieve stillness and clarity; to generate a strong, healthy, disease-free body; and to maintain internal balance while either your inner world or the events of the external world are rapidly changing.

Longevity Breathing Yoga

Taoist yoga is ancient China's soft yet powerful alternative to what is popularly known today as hatha yoga. The system Frantzis has developed to teach China's yoga is called Longevity Breathing® yoga. Its primary emphasis is to stimulate the flow of chi and free blocked energy. Combining gentle postures and Longevity Breathing techniques systematically opens the body's energy channels, thereby activating and stimulating chi flow. Postures, held from two to five minutes, require virtually no muscular effort. This lets you easily focus on what is internal so you can feel where the chi is blocked and gently free it up.

Healing Others with Qigong Tui Na

Part of Frantzis' Taoist training was to become a Chinese doctor, primarily using the qigong healing techniques known as qigong tui na. During this training period, he worked with more than 10,000 patients. Frantzis no longer works as a qigong doctor, either privately or in clinics, but occasionally offers training in therapeutic healing techniques.

Qigong tui na is a special branch of Chinese medicine that is designed to unblock, free and balance chi in others. You learn to project energy from your hands, voice and eyes to facilitate healing using 200 hand techniques. You also learn how to avoid burnout from your therapeutic practice. To heal others, you must first learn to unblock and free your own chi and to control the specific pathways through which it flows.

Shengong

Whereas *chi* (or *qi*) means "energy," *shen* means "spirit." Spirit equals meditation, which equals spirituality. So the term *shengong* literally means "spirit work."

Chi practices can make your body healthier and physically stronger. Meditation is about going beyond the energy of your flesh and internal organs where the primal or instinctual emotions reside. In terms of meditation, shengong is the fusion of qigong with the emotional, mental, psychic and karmic energy bodies to the level of your essence. This is the point at which you move into Taoist meditation.

Taoist Meditation

Frantzis is a lineage holder in the gentle Water method of Taoist meditation passed down from the teachings of Lao Tse over 2,500 years ago. Taoist meditation is little known in the West and is often confused with Buddhism. In Taoism, the road to spirituality involves more than having health, calmness and a stable, peaceful mind. These are just the necessary prerequisites and are achieved through qigong, Longevity Breathing, tai chi and other Taoist energy programs.

Taoist meditation includes using chi to help you release anxieties, expectations, and negative emotions—referred to as blockages—that prevent you from feeling truly alive and joyful. The first goal is to address spiritual responsibility for yourself, helping you become a relaxed, spontaneous, fully mature and open human being. A second goal is awakening the great human potential inside you, fostering compassion and balance. The third is reaching inner stillness—a place deep inside you that is absolutely permanent and stable. As your practice deepens, the sixteen-part neigong system is brought into play to accelerate the evolutionary spiritual process.

Training Opportunities

Bruce Frantzis is the founder of Energy Arts, Inc. which is based in Marin County, California. Energy Arts offers instructor certification programs, retreats, corporate and public workshops and lectures worldwide. Frantzis teaches Energy Arts courses in qigong; Longevity Breathing; the internal martial arts of bagua and tai chi; Longevity Breathing yoga; the healing techniques of qigong tui na; and Taoist meditation.

Instructor Certification

Prior training in Frantzis Energy Arts programs is a requirement for most instructor courses. The certification process is rigorous to ensure that instructors teach the authentic traditions inherent in these arts.

Train with a Certified Instructor

EnergyArts.com contains a directory of all Frantzis Certified Instructors worldwide. Since Frantzis no longer offers regular ongoing classes, he recommends locating an instructor in your area for regular training and for building on or preparing for his teachings.

Contact Information

Energy Arts, Inc.
P. O. Box 99
Fairfax, CA 94978-0099 USA
Phone: 415.454.5243
Fax: 415.454.0907

We invite you to visit EnergyArts.com to:

- Sign up for free monthly articles by Bruce Frantzis

- Receive the latest details on events and training materials

- Discover ways to join us in addressing the health crisis

- Watch video clips of qigong and martial arts forms

- Find a Certified Instructor near you or learn how to become one

- Inquire about hosting a workshop or speaking engagement.

BIBLIOGRAPHY

Chuang Tzu, *The Way of Chuang Tzu,* translated by Thomas Merton. Shambhala Publications, 2004.

The Bible, Genesis 2:7

Lao Tse (Lao Tzu), *Tao Te Ching,* various English translations available.

Lipton, Bruce H., *The Biology of Belief: Unleashing the Power of Consciousness, Matter and Miracles.* Mountain of Love Productions and Elite Press, 2005.

McTaggart, Lynne, *The Intention Experiment: Using Your Thoughts to Change Your Life and the World.* Free Press, a division of Simon & Schuster, Inc., 2007.

McTaggart, Lynne, *The Field: The Quest for the Secret Force of the Universe.* Harper Paperbacks, an imprint of HarperCollins Publishers, 2003.

The Original I Ching Oracle, translated by Rudolf Ritsema and Shantena Augusto Sabbadini. Watkins Publishing, 2005.

Zhuangzi (Chuang Tzu) *Zhuangzi: Basic Writings,* translated by Burton Watson. Columbia University Press, 2003.